Cheeseburger Pneumonia
...and other Surgery Stories

Anthony M. Rizzo, M.D.
Colonel (Ret.) USAF, MC, SFS

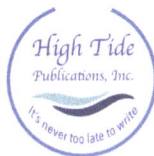

High Tide
Publications, Inc.
It's never too late to write

Published by High Tide Publications, Inc.
Deltaville, Virginia
www.Hightidepublications.com

Thank you for choosing this authorized edition of *Cheeseburger Pneumonia... And Other Surgery Stories*. At High Tide, our mission is to discover, promote, and publish the work of talented authors over 50. Your support by purchasing an authorized copy is crucial in helping us bring their work to you.

Your support in our mission to bring the work of our authors to a wider audience is deeply appreciated. Thank you for choosing to purchase an authorized edition.

Edited by Cindy L. Freeman (cindylfreeman.com)
Book design by Jeanne Johansen

First edition December, 2025

Printed in the United States of America.

To my wife and children

You've certainly put up with a LOT

Contents

Introduction

This is a book of surgery stories. It is not my life story.

I am frequently irritated when I pick up a book whose title proclaims to tell a particular story, only to find I must wade through the protagonist's childhood, first broken heart, etc. before I can get to the meat advertised in the title.

So, you're not going to read about my childhood poverty or abusive father. Not going to read about my being the first in the family to go to college, much less medical school. Not going to read about how I managed to get through school by working full-time. Not going to read about my mother's death during my freshman year of medical school and the profound impact that had on me. Not going to read about my time in the U.S. Public Health Service. Not going to read about my time in the Central Intelligence Agency as an undercover intelligence officer or how my cover was blown, and I was moved to the U.S. Air Force. Not going to read about my time working for Walt Disney World (but if you want to read about that, please get *Doctor to the Mouse: Stories from a Walt Disney World Physician* available on Amazon.com). Not going to read about 9/11, my directing the Surgeon General's Think Tank for Homeland Defense, then being a plank holder at U.S. Northern Command. Not going to read about my becoming the director of the Armed Forces Medical Intelligence Center. Not going to read about my directorship of the National Center for Medical Intelligence under the auspices of the Defense Intelligence Agency. Not going to read about my becoming a professor of anatomy and physiology at a state college.

Nope. You're not going to read about any of that.

You're just going to read stories about surgery, as an important part of my life was my practice of general surgery in both the Air Force and the civilian world.

I have always thought, and used to say whenever I was in a group of surgeons, that surgery is a specialty filled with sociopaths who have found a legal and socially acceptable way to exist in society. I loved to poke the bear.

"What do you mean by that, Rizzo?" would be the huffy response from other surgeons.

"Think about it," I'd answer. "Surgeons work hard to control feelings of tension in their lives until the morning they can scrub into the OR. There, they inflict a deadly wound on a helpless victim and root around the victim's insides. What they do in the OR would be a crime anywhere else. After closing the victim, the surgeon feels relief, satisfaction, and maybe a little controlled euphoria. Doesn't that sound like a sociopath prior to, during, and after committing antisocial behavior?"

I was never well liked among my fellow surgeons.

I have purposely not identified my medical school, my residency, or the names of the characters in this book, because a lot of these stories are indictments of institutions or persons. If you recognize yourself in this book, I hope you're doing better now.

Please know that the medical school and residency environments I describe in this book are "then," not "now." Then, we had a quota for the number of women in the class. My medical school class was ten percent women. Now, over fifty percent of medical students are female.

While I am not affiliated with a medical school, and cannot say for certain how things are currently run, I am confident that students do not practice procedures on each other as we did. I know that both medical students and residents are limited in the number of hours they can work before being given a rest—although I don't know how well that is enforced.

When I was in training, we worked day and night to the point of exhaustion and, sometimes, to the point of the psychotic behavior that comes with sleep deprivation.

Practice has also changed significantly. My days would start with morning rounds on my inpatients—patients I had operated on. If it was a clinic day, I would then spend the day seeing patients in the clinic, followed by evening rounds on my inpatients. Since I operated on the patients, the philosophy was I was also completely responsible for their pre-op and post-op care. Thus, at all times of the day and night, the nurses would call with questions or input about my inpatients. On an operating day the OR substituted for the clinic, while the inpatients still had to be attended to. On on-call days the ER was added to the above.

When one of my inpatients required a consult from a different specialty, such as pulmonology or cardiology, I always wrote, "Consultant not to write orders until discussed with me." I was in charge of the total care of my patients, and that was the prevailing practice for every physician who admitted patients.

Today, admitting a patient means turning that patient over to a hospitalist. Doctors don't know what happened to their patient until they read the discharge summary.

Thankfully, medicine and surgery have changed from the '70s and '80s. This is how it was then…

Medical School

"The road to the operating room is paved with sleepless nights, missed meals, and the humbling realization that you do not know everything. But it leads to the only place where you can holda human heart in your hands and give it a second chance."

— Unknown (Common Medical School Adage)

My First Surgery

How did he get a fork up his ass?

Let's find out...

The third year of medical school was where we were put on the wards of the hospital and asked to see patients. It was immediately apparent we were woefully unprepared.

The third year was divided into rotations. Three months of internal medicine. Three months of surgery. Three months of pediatrics. Six weeks of obstetrics and gynecology. Six weeks of psychiatry. There were no breaks or vacations. We were in the hospital every day, and we were on call every third night.

On call meant you worked all day, were up all night, then worked all the next day. There were no set hours when you went home. You went home when the work was done. The work was never done.

My first day of surgery rotation happened to also be my first night on call in surgery. Ed was the senior resident. I had no idea what I was doing, but Ed was a fifth-year surgery resident in a seven-year residency. He had every idea what he was doing—thank goodness—and took pity on me.

He got called to the ER for a surgical consult, then paged me to meet him on the ward. He had admitted an elderly man who had a perirectal abscess.

A perirectal abscess is a collection of pus immediately adjacent to the anus. Because it is the result of an infection from bacteria that originated in the colon, there is a real risk of a patient with a perirectal abscess becoming septic.

Sepsis is the number one cause of death in ICUs in the United States, so it is nothing to take lightly.

Of course, I didn't realize any of that at the time. I was just blunderingly following where Ed told me to go and doing what Ed told me to do.

Ed told me we were going to the operating room to incise and drain (I&D) the abscess.

Wow! My first day on surgery, my first night on call, and I was going to the OR!

I was clueless as to how to do that.

Ed took me to the surgeon's changing room, showed me where to get scrubs, and how to get a locker for my clothes.

Side note: unlike today, where it seems everyone in the hospital wears scrubs, when I was in medical school only surgeons wore scrubs. And scrubs were only to be worn in the OR. My uniform was white pants, a shirt and tie, and a short white coat. The short coat indicated I was a medical student. Our tie clips were plastic with our names engraved on them. When we were first years, each med school year was issued a different color tie clip. My year was yellow. That was how the hospital staff knew who was who and could make a pretty good guess at our level of ignorance.

Ed patiently showed me how to do a ten-minute scrub from hands to elbows, then how to remain sterile and enter the OR without contaminating myself, him, the nurses, or the surgical instruments. He showed me how to gown and glove, again avoiding contaminating everyone and everything in the room.

The patient was already in the OR, since Ed and I had placed him there on the operating table prior to scrubbing our hands and forearms. After he was asleep, the patient was placed in the lithotomy position.

The lithotomy position is named for the lithotomy procedure. Lithotomy is based on Greek for stone removal. Once upon a time bladder stones were common, and patients were placed in the lithotomy position so someone could put a sound (a metal rod) into their bladder through their urethra to try to break up the stones. It is as awful as it sounds, especially without anesthesia.

Women are placed in the lithotomy position to have a pelvic exam.

So, this patient was on his back with his lower extremities up in stirrups and his butt hanging off the end of the OR table.

He had a huge, red, inflamed abscess immediately to the left of his anus.

After prepping the area with surgical soap, Ed incised and drained the abscess. That means he took a knife and stabbed the abscess, draining the pus inside.

It seemed like gallons of pus, blood, and stool came rolling out of this abscess. The smell was overpowering. Then the tine of a plastic fork fell out of the wound. I asked Ed how the fork tine could have gotten there. Ed just laughed.

After packing the wound, leaving it open, and giving the patient a dressing, we took him to the recovery room.

The next morning, on rounds, Ed asked the patient about the plastic fork tine.

The patient was surprised we would not know how it got there.

He stated he had been constipated, so he took a plastic fork, inserted it into his anus and rectum, and attempted to dig the impacted stool from his rectal vault. He guessed one of the tines must have broken off.

It would have been nice if the patient had told us about his putting a fork up his rectum pre-op. But he didn't. So, we didn't know until then what had caused the abscess. The patient had perforated his rectum with the fork, broken off a tine, and introduced stool and rectal bacteria into the tissue surrounding his rectum.

Pus, blood, stool, a mysterious plastic fork tine, and an unforgettable smell defined the first surgery I had ever seen. It was quite the introduction to what would become my specialty. But at the time I didn't know that. I intended to be a family physician…

Over the years, I realized I had learned quite a lot from this case. Not the least of the lessons was that patients almost never tell you the whole story. And the part of the story patients will tell you is frequently, frequently, frequently false.

What Was Medical School Like?

When I attended medical school, between 1972 and 1977, U.S. medicine was male-dominated. My medical school class had a quota of ten females out of a class of 100. Of those ten, one committed suicide via carbon monoxide poisoning. One quit in the first year and became a waitress. One, the only African American woman in the class, died that first year of ovarian cancer. Of the other African American students in the class, several had been admitted under affirmative action criteria and were not academically qualified, thus they either dropped out or failed out in the first year.

We were a bunch of lily-white males.

Except for one of my partners, a female who had been a biochemistry major in college. She was a driven person who had sacrificed everything of her typical development to get into medical school. For example, she was still a virgin. She begged another of my classmate partners to sleep with her because she wanted to experience sex—once—so that she could relate to future patients. Sadly, she also committed suicide later in life.

The school had virtually no idea what to do with, or how to treat, the women in our class. One of the most egregious examples of the thoughtless way the females were treated had to do with how we were taught various procedures.

We learned them on each other.

We started IVs on each other. We passed nasogastric tubes on each other (tubes that were inserted into the nose, down the esophagus, and into the stomach).

We sigmoidoscoped each other.

One morning in the first year, the class was divided into pairs, and each pair was given a sigmoidoscope.

A sigmoidoscope is an approximately two-foot-long rigid metal tube that is inserted into the anus and up into the rectum and sigmoid colon (S-shaped last part of the large intestine). This allows physicians to look at the inside of the colon.

Fred, Elliot, and Penny, my anatomy partners, were my partners in this exercise, as well. I was paired with Elliot and Fred was paired with Penny.

One of us had the sigmoidoscope and the other was to be examined.

In turns, one of us was to pull down our pants and underwear and bend over a classroom table. The other was to put the scope into our partner's rectum and look around. The fact that we were a bunch of men with a few women in the class, and that none of us really wanted to disrobe, much less be scoped in front of each other, was simply ignored.

"Get on with it!" was the instruction from our professors.

Penny dutifully pulled down her pants and panties and bent over a table. Fred lubricated the scope and inserted it into Penny's large intestine.

Penny was a person who blushed easily. Fred knew this and habitually told obscene jokes to make Penny blush.

Once Fred had the scope in Penny's colon, he told one of his more obscene jokes. Penny blushed.

"Hey, everyone!" yelled Fred. "When Penny blushed her colon blushed, too! Come and look!"

It is the case that the nerves that cause blood vessels in the skin to dilate and make you blush do the same with the lining of the intestines. We learned that bit of anatomy and physiology that morning when every one of us came over and looked into Penny's rectum.

But then Fred withdrew and cleaned the scope, and Penny got to scope

Fred. She was none too gentle.

Side note: I'm pretty sure this kind of instruction is no longer happening in medical schools. Sigmoidoscopy is probably taught with a mannequin. Med students aren't required to disrobe in front of each other, much less practice procedures on each other. I'm sure there's some education in today's method, but the students lose knowing how it feels to have a procedure performed on them, and they also would not learn about blushing colons!

This being the 1970s, things were fast and loose when it came to supervising medical students, interns, and residents. There was very little supervision. We were expected to learn by doing. See one, do one, teach one was the rule of the day. It was not until my chief resident year in 1989 (there was a long delay between my internship and my residency while I worked for the CIA—another story) that the first laws requiring sleep were passed. More on that later....

For my entire training I was on call either every third or every other night. If every third, that meant working all day starting at 5:00 am, being up and working all night, working the next day until the work was done (the work was never done) going home around 8 or 9:00 pm, working the next day from 5:00 am until 8 or 9:00 pm, then starting the three-day cycle again.

If you were on a rotation that was every other day on call, you worked from 5:00 am through that day and night and the next day, got off around 9:00 pm, then started the next morning at 5:00 am to do it all again.

It was brutal.

In the surgery residency the question was asked, "What is the problem with being on call every other night?" The answer? "You miss half of the cases."

Seeing attendings (our teachers) was rare on some rotations, never on others, and, sometimes, you might see an attending for a short time during the day. So, who was teaching us? If we were a third-year student, we were taught by a fourth-year student, an intern, or a resident. Who was teaching them? Another resident just above them, but also still in training.

Mistakes

D id we make mistakes?
Yes.

A lot of mistakes.

This is a book about surgery stories, but here's one on me that was medical to show you what I mean about lack of supervision and learning by doing:

My first third-year rotation was internal medicine. That meant, after two years of classroom instruction, I was put on a medicine team and expected to take care of critically sick hospital patients with medical problems. I was on call every third night when on that rotation.

I didn't have a clue about what I was doing.

One evening about 6:00 pm, after working since 5:00 am, I was on call and on the ward with a second-year medicine resident and a medical intern. The resident said to me, "There's a patient in room 403 bed A who's not making any urine. I need you to get him to pee."

"How do I do that?" I asked.

"Give him some Lasix®," he said.

"How much?" I asked.

"Look it up!" I had exhausted his patience by asking those two questions. He disappeared, not to be seen until morning.

I turned to the intern. He looked at me and started to say something, but his pager went off. He was called to the ER, not to be seen until the morning.

At the nursing station on each ward there was a book: the Physician's Desk Reference or PDR. It was hundreds of pages of small print describing every medication there was. Today it's on everyone's phone as an app. But I trained before the internet and before computers.

I looked up Lasix®. Lasix® had a lot of pages about it, but I wasn't about to spend twenty minutes reading all of that. I had to get this guy to pee, plus all the other work I had to do that had been assigned when the team made evening rounds. So, I only read the part about dosage and administration.

It said to start with 20mg IV, then double that dose if there was no effect.

That's all I read.

I got the chart for the man in 403 bed A and wrote an order for 20mg of Lasix® IV push. I didn't bother to read the rest of the chart.

Of course, the nurses were not stupid. They would never take off an order written by a medical student that hadn't been co-signed by an RD (real doctor).

Side note: taking off an order meant reading the order in the chart then transcribing it to whomever needed to follow the order, such as the pharmacy, X-ray, or the other nurses.

That meant I now became the nurse for this patient. I took off the order myself, which meant tearing off the pharmacy copy of the order sheet—the order sheet was a triplicate form. Remember, there were no computers.

I then put the pharmacy copy in the pneumatic tube that sent the order down to the pharmacy. After a while the tube delivered a syringe with 20mg of Lasix®.

I took the syringe and marched into 403, bed A, to get my first look at the patient.

He was an elderly African American man, sleeping with the sheet pulled over his head. A foley catheter protruded from under the side of the sheet to an empty foley bag. Yup, this guy was not making any urine.

Side note: my hospital was a huge public city hospital in the Midwest that had a large African American population. Almost all the patients were indigent African Americans. Today, our lack of supervision when learning on these people would be considered racist—and rightly so.

I had no idea if you pushed Lasix quickly or slowly. I hadn't read that part. So, I guessed and pushed it "medium" into the piggyback port of the man's IV line. I at least had the decency to tell him what I was doing, but I had to awaken him to do that. The fact that he was sleeping in the early evening didn't register on me as a problem I should think or worry about.

I stood at the bedside for a couple of minutes staring at the foley tube and bag. No urine. How long was I supposed to wait? I hadn't read that part. But I was in a hurry. I had lots of work to do. And I had to make this man pee.

So, I went back to the nursing station and wrote an order for 40mg of Lasix®. I took off the order, tubed it down, waited, and got back a syringe with 40mg of Lasix®. Which I again pushed "medium." With no result.

Did I bother to call the intern and ask what I should do? The resident? Nope. They were busy and had told me to do this job. I was not about to suffer the indignity and verbal abuse that would have accompanied asking them a question.

How about the nurses? Did I ask a nurse—who most certainly would have known the answer? Nope.

I was a medical student!!! I was never going to debase myself by asking a nurse a question.

And the nurses were smart enough to stay out of the medical students' ways. The nurses had learned long ago that we were a bunch of egotistical assholes.

Instead, I wrote an order for another doubling of the Lasix® dose, took it off, sent it down, got it back, and administered 80mg of Lasix®

Then 160mg.

Then 320mg.

Then 640mg.

Then 1,280mg.

In total I gave the poor victim of my ignorance and pride 2,540mg of Lasix® IV push over a period of a couple of hours.

The man was very lucky, because it turns out Lasix® is relatively safe. Relatively. There are many untoward effects of too much Lasix®. But I didn't know any of that.

Low and behold, a few cc's of dark yellow urine trickled out of the foley tube and into the bag.

So, my work was done.

I spent the rest of the night doing what third-year med students did, and probably still do: started IVs, changed dressings, etc.

At 5:00 am, the intern and resident showed up on the ward. They had been up all night working in either the ER or another part of the hospital. We had to make our rounds to prepare for rounding again with the attending who was due at 8:00 am.

"Well, Rizzo, did you get the guy in 403 to pee?" asked the resident.

"Yup. Sure did."

"What?! How did you do that?"

I told him.

"Rizzo, didn't you read the chart?"

"No…"

"If you had read the chart, you would have known that man is in complete renal failure. He is due for his first dialysis this morning."

"Then why did you tell me to get him to pee?" I asked.

"I was joking! If you had read the chart, you would have known that!"

"Oh."

"When the attending shows up, I want you to keep your mouth shut. Don't say a word. Don't answer a question, even if he asks you directly."

"OK."

It never occurred to me that the resident was going to have to cosign my stupid, ignorant orders after the fact. Meaning, if there was a long-term complication of my actions, he would be responsible.

But it taught me to read the charts and ask questions if I didn't know what I was doing.

So, I guess I learned something. Too bad I learned it—like we all learned so many things during our unsupervised training—at the expense of my patient.

Praying to God

To give you an idea of what our medical school was like in 1972, here is a picture of the gross (as opposed to microscopic) anatomy lab:

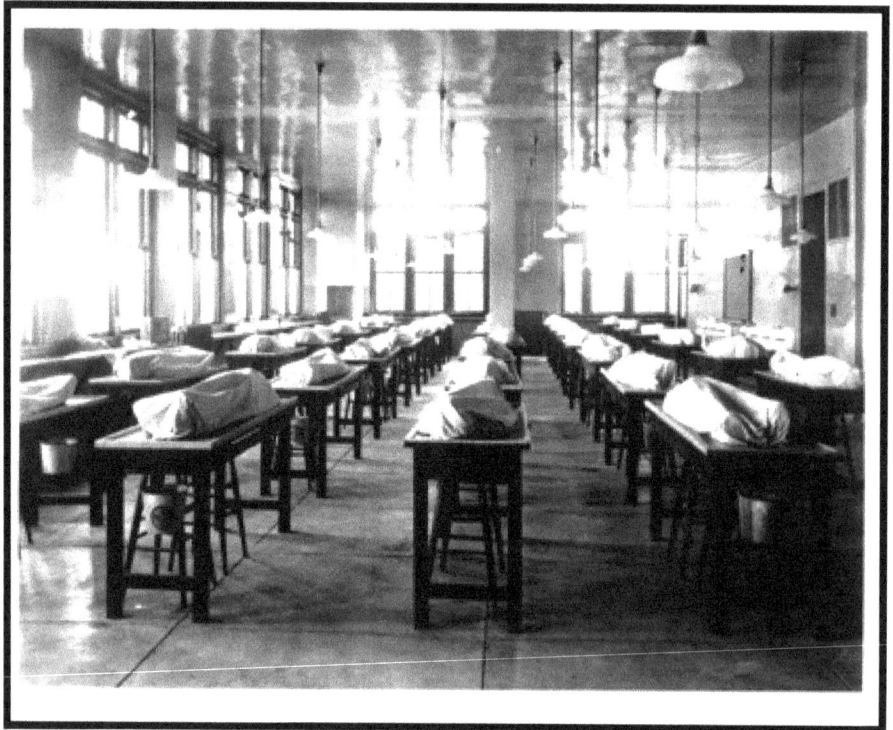

Gross Anatomy Lab

Each of those tables held a cadaver. Unlike today, where medical school cadavers for dissection and learning anatomy are almost exclusively from donors, our cadavers were primarily from indigent people experiencing homelessness whose dead bodies went unclaimed.

The lab was neither heated nor air conditioned. It was brutally hot in the summer, so we opened the windows. Hello, flies!

It was brutally cold in the winter, so we wore coats under our dissecting gowns.

We were divided into groups of four students per cadaver. Those four students became partners in almost every class during the first two pre-clinical years. My partners were—and this is relevant—Fred, Elliot, and Penny. Fred was a registered nurse who had been a comparative religion major in college. He was the only RN in our class, as medical schools almost never accept nurses. Fred was Jewish by birth but was a devout agnostic. Elliot was one of the few married students in our class, which is why we never went to his house to study. Elliot was also a devout Jew. Penny had been a biochemistry major in college and was what was called a gunner in medical school. A gunner is the person who studies incessantly and always knows the answer to any question a professor might ask. Penny was a devout, practicing Catholic.

Besides anatomy, one of our first-year classes was biochemistry. Of course, Penny had been a biochem major, was a gunner, and was fully expected by the rest of our little group to ace the biochem final.

That is an important point, as we only had one exam in biochem—the final. Students either passed that test and stayed in medical school, or they didn't and failed out completely. Fred had no interest whatsoever in biochemistry. He didn't study during the entire quarter. Penny kept nagging him, but Fred just ignored both her and biochemistry.

Our school didn't have grades. It was a pass/fail system. Well, not quite. The school gave out Honors, High Pass, Pass, Low Pass, and Fail. Sounded like A, B, C, D, F to us, but the administrators insisted it was just pass/fail.

The week before the big biochem final Fred began to panic. He said to Penny, "What do I have to do to pass this class?"

Penny replied, "You have no chance of passing this class. You haven't studied all quarter. But I will study with you every day and night for this week before the test and hopefully you can eke out a low pass."

That is exactly what happened. Penny drilled Fred on biochem day and night for a week.

The night before the test the four of us were together, studying in Fred's apartment. Since Penny had the apartment next to Fred's, they had literally spent an entire week together mired in biochemistry. Fred asked Penny, "Do I have a chance tomorrow?"

Penny answered, "You have no chance whatsoever. The only chance you have is this: I am going to pray to God tonight to help you pass the test. If you pass, it will be a miracle from God." Remember, Fred was an agnostic, so this was not exactly reassuring him.

The next day we all took the biochem final. It was brutal.

Several days later the grades were posted. Literally. On a bulletin board were our names and grades for all to see.

Penny, whom we all expected to get an Honors, got a Pass.

Fred, whom we all expected to fail, got an Honors.

Penny was disappointed in her own grade—we knew it couldn't be correct—but she was ecstatic for Fred. "Fred, God worked a miracle. That is the only way you could have gotten an Honors!" Penny felt that God had answered her prayer.

Two days later, we were all standing around our cadaver, dissecting, when one of the deans came into the lab and walked up to our table. "Fred, I need to see you," he said. The dean took Fred out of the lab. This was an unheard-of event. Not only did our table stop dissecting, but the tables all around ours stopped. What could this mean? We all felt in our bones that whatever it meant, it couldn't be good.

One of the students at the table next to ours had a last name that was alphabetically next to Fred's on the grade list. This guy was also a gunner. He was also an ass. He had gotten a Low Pass on the biochem test and was whining, long and loud, about the injustice of him getting a Low Pass when Fred got an Honors. This guy had fully expected Honors and was seemingly never going to shut up about it.

Fred returned. It seems that Fred's grade and the grade of the gunner next to us had been switched accidentally. Fred was told his true grade was Low Pass.

Of course, when we heard this, we all assumed, and said out loud, that we were pretty sure Fred had failed the test but that the school was too embarrassed to change his grade from Honors to Fail. We all thought, and said, that Fred's Low Pass was a gift.

Fred had only this to say, "Penny, God is an Indian giver." Yes, I know this is now considered racist....

The Magic Forceps

Constantly circulating through the anatomy lab was one of the medical school deans, Dr. A, who was also a professor of anatomy. He carried in the breast pocket of his lab coat "The Magic Forceps." We might dissect for an hour trying to find a particular structure and never find it. In frustration, we would call Dr. A over, knowing what was to happen. He would whip The Magic Forceps out of his pocket and use it to instantly point out the elusive structure. Then we would be subjected to a dose of verbal abuse and condescension that none of us relished.

Two tables over from ours was a male cadaver that had, because of the embalming technique used on him, an erection.

One day that team of medical students had had enough of the professor, his Magic Forceps, and his condescending attitude.

They folded the erect penis down and covered it with their heavy, brown rubberized fabric cadaver cover.

Then they raised their collective hands and waited for Dr. A to stroll over, which he did with a patronizing grin.

"Dr. A, we've been looking for an hour. We can't find the ovaries."

Dr. A's grin grew wider in anticipation of the load of abuse he was about to heap upon that team.

Dr. A whipped out his Magic Forceps, bent over the cadaver, and hesitated. Next, Dr. A started to move pelvic organs around. Then he asked for a scissor and started to dissect.

Dr. A spent well over five minutes looking for the non-existent ovaries. By this time, pretty much all the med school class had gathered around that table.

Then Dr. A looked up. He did not have the condescending grin on his face. He saw the entire class grouped around him.

Realization dawned. He reached down, threw back the rubberized cloth cover, and we all watched as the penis erected from between the cadaver's thighs.

The class burst out laughing. Dr. A did not join in. He silently put his Magic Forceps into his breast pocket and left the lab.

To pass anatomy we had both written and oral exams. Each quarter there was a single oral exam held at the cadaver—one professor grilling a med student team for one hour.

Guess which professor gave the exam to the team with the elusive ovaries?

Sex Ed

To give you another idea about how our medical education went in the 1970s, let me tell you about sex education week.

Between the first and second years of medical school we had a summer break, like the kind of summer break seen in high school and college. There was no such break between the second and third years or between the third and fourth years. Once we started the second year, it was full speed ahead until graduation.

We all got a letter during that summer between the first and second years mandating us to return to campus one week early. No reason for this was given. The letter only said that attendance was required, and we were to assemble in the auditorium at 8:00 am on the first day back.

So, we all changed our plans and showed up a week early.

When we got to the auditorium, a significant number of faculty were assembled on the stage. One of the professors came forward from that august group and said, "Until now, this medical school has not taught anything about human sexuality during the four years of medical school training. Yours is to be the first class to receive instruction in human sexuality. You will report to this auditorium at 8:00 am each morning this week, you will get instruction, then you will be broken into small groups from 9:00 until noon. At noon you will go to lunch. At 1:00 pm you will reassemble here in the auditorium for instruction, then back to small groups until 5:00 pm."

He went on to say that, because the school had never taught human sexuality before, the faculty was not sure how to go about it. But they had been meeting all summer and had decided we were likely to laugh, be shocked, or be embarrassed by the instruction. So, to desensitize us to the subject, we would watch pornography for one hour each day at both 8:00 am and 1:00 pm.

Oh. My. God.

That is exactly what they did. It was appalling.

But that was nothing compared to the Friday afternoon session. After the mandatory pornography, we were kept in the auditorium. On the stage appeared an elderly professor and three women. The professor stated these were prostitutes—his words—he had picked up from the street in his car during the lunch hour. He was paying them to be on the stage and answer any questions we might have.

You could have heard a pin drop. No one could believe what he had said. We all looked at those poor women and could not imagine what they must be thinking. These women were abused by men for a living. Now they were on a stage, under lights, looking at a room full of men (and seven women) who were silently staring at them.

We had no questions.

The professor ranted at us. "Open your mouths and ask something!"

No one spoke.

The women on stage were obviously very uncomfortable with this situation.

Finally, as none of us opened our mouths, the professor became angry and, yelling, dismissed us.

I assume he gave those poor women a ride back downtown to where he had picked them up.

We all wondered what would have happened if he had been arrested for soliciting.

But at least we got an early afternoon off.

Suture Doctor

During my first and second years as a medical student, I had a job as a suture doctor in the city hospital's ER. Being a suture doctor is something that would never happen today, but at the time I was in medical school the rules were, as previously mentioned, a little loose as compared to now. Without any training at all, medical students were hired to suture lacerations. We learned on the job, meaning we learned on injured humans. And we didn't have YouTube to watch.

I found a book, talked to some of the other suture doctors, and asked a surgery resident for some instructions. But I got precious little instruction. I just started to work.

Because I was in the ER so often, I got to see an enormous amount of human pathology even though I was a lowly first- and second-year medical student.

Every second or third day, the police would bring in a woman named AW. AW was a homeless woman who lived under one of the viaducts in the downtown area. She was a serious alcoholic. The police always brought her in because she was unconscious on the street under her viaduct.

Every time she was brought in, she was placed in one of the first two rooms, which were dedicated to triage. An emergency medicine resident, usually a second-year in a three-year program (I never, ever saw an ER attending in the ER) would enter the triage room, take a look at AW from as far away as possible, declare her stable, and tell the nurses to put her in the back hall (no ER staff ever went into the back hall). Admittedly, AW was filthy, had usually soiled herself with feces, and smelled truly awful.

And, since this was a repeat performance with a known outcome, the residents felt secure just placing AW in the back hall without much more than a cursory glance.

The performance I am referring to is this: when AW woke up from her alcohol-induced stupor, she would start screaming at the top of her lungs. If anyone was within range of her upper or lower extremities, he or she could 100% count on being slugged or kicked. If within range of her head, one could count on being bitten. She was also known to smear feces on her gurney, the walls, or people within reach. She would then get off the gurney and walk out of the hospital.

AW was a "frequent flyer." The residents, who had seen her repeatedly for as long as anyone could remember, felt confident she was never in any acute distress, so they never examined AW.

One day while I was working in the suture room, AW came in again, unconscious as usual, and smelling terrible as usual. The second-year ER resident glanced at her from the door of the triage room, pronounced her stable, and sentenced her to the back hall. As usual.

Sometime later, I was walking through the back hall and looked over at AW. She was still unconscious long after the amount of time it usually took for her to wake up, scream, and leave.

I got a little closer and noticed AW did not appear to be breathing. I felt for a pulse in her neck. There was no pulse.

AW was dead.

I hurriedly called the ER resident. He walked back, took a look, and became worried very quickly. It was his signature on the chart, a chart that said she had been evaluated and was stable to be in the back hall.

But AW was not coded (meaning no one called the resuscitation team or tried to resuscitate her). No one started CPR. No one did anything except worry about what would happen to them because AW had died without being evaluated.

Even though I was a lowly medical student suture doctor, I suggested to the resident we get some X-rays on AW's body to see if we could figure out what killed her. We couldn't get any blood because she had been dead long enough to have clotted in her vessels.

An orderly wheeled AW from the back hall into ER X-ray where she got abdominal and chest films and a cross-table lateral of her neck.

AW had a broken neck. Her broken neck caused her to stop breathing and killed her.

Lesson learned? Perhaps the lesson is to always examine your patients. Or, perhaps, it is not to falsify charts and state you have examined someone you have not. Or, perhaps, it is not to be a frequent flyer.

***

One evening I was working in the suture room when I was given a patient who had walked through a plate glass sliding porch door. He had lacerations everywhere.

He was handcuffed to the stretcher and had a police escort.

He was on PCP (a potent hallucinogen) and had decided he was Jesus.

And he was one of my classmates.

It was horrible to see him in that state. He was clearly under PCP's influence, with grandiose speech and hallucinations. He tried to verbally "cast me out" when I approached the stretcher.

When I gave him a tetanus shot in his shoulder, he turned his head and puffed on the syringe in the belief he could stop the injection.

I sutured him up and sent him off with the police.

It was the last time we saw him at the medical school.

It was also the first—but not the last—time a patient brought me to tears.

CT Scanner

While I was a third-year medical student, our city general hospital took delivery of the first CT scanner in the United States. CT (Computed Tomography) scanners are X-ray machines that deliver three-dimensional views of the inside of the body.

Everyone was excited! What were we going to be able to do? The hype was that we would be able to see everything inside a patient! No more having to take people to the OR to open their abdomen or chest and explore them! Just run them through the CT!

The trouble was that no one had ever seen a CT image. No one knew what we would be able to see. There was no library of normal anatomy as seen by the scanner.

Radiology wanted to build a library of "normals" with which to compare findings in disease.

While I was on my pediatric rotation, a child—let's call him P—was born to consanguineous parents. P was anencephalic. P's parents were a severely mentally challenged brother and sister who were institutionalized together in a state facility. The state had a policy to sterilize institutionalized females at menarche (first menstrual period), but this young person fell through the cracks. Her brother impregnated her.

An anencephalic child is born without a cerebral cortex. Such children have a brainstem, so they can breathe, have a heartbeat, and have basic physiology in their organs. But they don't physically have any higher brain.

They can never think or even be conscious. These children almost always have additional physical abnormalities, frequently with abnormal hearts, kidneys, and other organs. Typically, such infants do not live long.

Because P was the product of consanguineous, mentally challenged, institutionalized parents, he was made a ward of the court.

The CT was due to be received about six months after P was born. When radiology found out there was an anencephalic child born they rushed to the pediatric ICU (PICU) where the kid was and asked the team there to keep the child going for six months. This request was so radiology could get CT images of a normal anencephalic for the library. They felt such an image would be invaluable when teaching radiology residents.

"What do you suggest we do with P after you get your CT scan?" asked the pediatric residents.

"Normally he would die anyway, so just let him die," was the radiologists' answer.

Keeping P going for six months would be a monumental task. He would be intubated, on a ventilator, fed by IVs and a feeding tube, and turned often to keep him from getting decubiti (bed sores). He was almost certain to get infected, probably multiple times, as well as develop pneumonia while on the ventilator. The hospital bill for all of this would, even back then, run into millions of dollars.

But, because there was also real value in getting a CT of his head, the pediatric department formally requested the court—P's legal parent—to rule on what to do.

Surprisingly, the court ruled that P was to be kept going so the CT could be obtained. The state would bear the cost of P's six-month hospitalization.

The question of P taking up a valuable and limited PICU bed, while certainly going to die, was also discussed but ignored by the court. Indeed, during that six months, there were times the bed was needed for a child who could live—but the bed was occupied by P.

Did P feel pain? Almost everything we did for him over the six months we awaited the CT scanner would hurt. P certainly had a brainstem, but did he have a limbic system, the part of the brain that receives pain signals?

We did not know, and, ironically, could not know if P had a limbic system without a CT scan! Even if P did have a limbic system, without a cerebrum he could not interpret what he was feeling as pain. But, really, no one knew what was in P's head without a CT.

Six months went by. The PICU nurses had all grown attached to P. The nurses continually called the doctors, stating P was moving or making sounds that caused the nurses to think he was "getting better." Going up to PICU to see P was heart wrenching.

Finally, the CT was installed. P got his CT. The scan went into the Radiology library and was shared across the country with any hospital that was receiving and installing CT scanners.

After the CT, P went back to the PICU. There, after six months of heroic effort to keep him going, P's IVs were discontinued, his feeding tube was pulled, and he was taken from the ventilator. Within minutes he was gone.

Did he die?

Not according to his parent: the court. The court ruled that, because P did not have a cerebrum, he was brain dead at birth. So, turning off all of P's support was not killing him, as he was already dead.

But it didn't feel like that to us who had kept him going.

It's Never Easy

While on my third-year Pediatric rotation we had a little girl on the ward who continues to haunt me, even after all these years. Not a surgical case, but, prior to antibiotics, she would have been a surgical case—she would have had an amputation. She taught me a lot about decision making.

The patient was a four-month-old who was the product of rape between cousins. She had multiple physical and mental disabilities and was a ward of the court. Prior to her admission she had been in an orphanage.

She was admitted for generalized sepsis from a bacterium called *serratia marcescens*. Serratia was not considered a pathogen in those days. It was a bacterium that had never been found to cause disease. In fact, in first-year microbiology class, serratia was smeared on the hands of two of my classmates on a Tuesday and all of us were cultured on that Thursday to demonstrate how infection can spread.

Side note: we all had serratia on our hands after two days of the first two students touching doorknobs, desktops, etc. It was an effective demonstration of the spread of infection.

This patient was septic and critically ill, and the only organism that was cultured from her blood was serratia. She was the world's first reported case of pathogenic serratia. Our best guess as to why this patient was so sick from serratia was that her immune system was impaired because of her multiple physical abnormalities.

Her "parent," the court, had ordered "all necessary treatment, including heroic measures" be administered to this child. The reason was that the court was aware of a family wanting to adopt the child, even given her multiple abnormalities. For there to be a family that wanted this child was nothing short of miraculous.

The family who wanted to adopt the patient had already applied for adoption, and the adoption was working its way through the system. We were told the patient's adoption was probably going to be final in approximately three months.

Along with this child's sepsis and multiple physical abnormalities she was mildly anemic. The anemia could have been a consequence of her sepsis, or it could have been that her bone marrow (where blood cells are made) harbored another of her abnormalities—we weren't sure.

Side note: The senior pediatric resident on the service was a third-year resident (in a three-year program), so he was just a few months short of graduation. I had never met anyone like him. He had an eidetic memory for the medical literature that he apparently constantly read. No matter what problem we were discussing on rounds, he was able to quote a journal article about the problem, to include the author and the journal's volume and issue numbers. It never failed. Of course, none of us could ever do the same thing. Except once. Once we had a patient who, it seemed, had been poisoned, which brought up a general discussion of poisoning. In college I had gotten a research grant and had published a paper entitled "Dimethyl Mercury in the Rat" in *Proceedings of the Western Pharmacological Society*. Of course, today, I cannot remember the volume or issue of that journal, but back then I could. I was able to emulate the resident when he asked a question about heavy metal poisoning. "In Volume X, Issue Y, of *Proceedings of the Western Pharmacological Society*, Rizzo discovered…" The rest of the medical students and junior residents went nuts. *No one* had ever quoted an article back to this senior resident. For a *brief*—and I need to emphasize *brief*—moment I was a star.

Back to the patient.

The senior resident quoted an article that said antibiotics may be less effective in a person who is anemic. The article was not definite. It only said that the antibiotics may be less effective. But the senior resident wanted to transfuse the patient to see if the antibiotics might become more effective. Why? Because the patient's infection was not responding well to the antibiotics. The antibiotics seemed to be working slowly. She was still extremely sick from her sepsis.

And the court had been clear: we were to use "all necessary treatment, including heroic measures."

However, the future adoptive parents were Jehovah's Witnesses. Jehovah's Witnesses are opposed to the use of blood or blood products. They believe that in the bible (Genesis 9:4, Leviticus 17:10, and Acts 15:29) Christians are instructed to neither accept nor donate blood.

But these people were not the patient's parents yet. The court was the parent. The court's orders were clear and, based upon the court's orders, we planned to transfuse her.

When the future adoptive parents—who had no legal standing at that time—were told we were going to transfuse, they stated if we gave the patient blood they would cancel the adoption.

Now we were in a quandary. We were under a court order to do everything possible so the child could be adopted. But if we followed the court's order and gave blood, there would be no more adoption.

The future adoptive parents spent vast amounts of time at the patient's bedside and always brought a new stuffed animal—always colored red—when they visited. The only time they weren't at the bedside was overnight.

Should we sneak some blood into the patient in the middle of the night? We considered it.

But this child had been on the ward for a long time. The nurses had formed emotional attachments to the kid and to the future adoptive family. It was a certainty one of the nurses would tell the family if we covertly transfused the child.

Also, the house staff and medical students had formed a bond with both the patient and the family. These were good people who wanted to take on the almost overwhelming responsibility of caring for the patient while giving her a family. We all wanted the patient and the family to finalize the adoption.

We wanted to respect the family's wishes. But we also were under a court order. And no one was sure transfusion would make much of a difference in this case. The transfusion idea was the result of the senior resident having read one paper that stated transfusion *might* help.

If the family cancelled the adoption, this patient would spend the rest of her life in an institution. Her multiple medical problems made her virtually unadoptable by anyone but this family.

The senior resident kept insisting we transfuse. He made it clear his motive was to see if the one paper he read was correct.

The nurses and the rest of the team were resisting giving the transfusion. We argued that mild anemia could be treated with iron supplements, although giving iron would take a long time to raise the blood count while transfusion would be immediate.

Finally, finally, an attending showed up. His word would be law. The senior resident presented the case to the attending and insisted on transfusion. A junior resident then presented the quandary about the future adoptive parents and the orders of the court.

I will never forget the look on the attending's face when he heard the rest of the story from the junior resident—the attending was used to hearing only from the senior resident and, invariably, approved of the senior resident's plans.

After considering for several moments, the attending ordered us to give iron and not to transfuse. He said he would contact the court if needed. He took responsibility—as he should have—and went against the wishes of the senior resident. That was a historic first.

Senior Electives

Our senior year in medical school was a year of electives. One elective I took was three months of family practice.

By the time I was in the elective, I had pretty much decided I was going to be a surgeon. But, for my entire life up to that point I had said I was going to be a family physician in a small town. This elective would be telling.

And telling, it was.

I was assigned to a family physician who had never had a medical student before. He had applied to the medical school for a student, I suppose, or maybe he responded to a call from the school for volunteers. In any case, I was the first. Let's call him FP.

FP's office was in a small town about one hour's drive from the city my medical school was in. From the outside, the office seemed quite large.

When I entered on Monday morning at 7 a.m., I introduced myself to the receptionist who took me back to FP's private office. It was like nothing I had ever seen—ever—in my life. It was huge. It was appointed with the most gaudy and expensive furniture and accoutrements imaginable. Quite a bit was gold-plated or maybe solid gold.

FP greeted me, then took me around to meet his six partners. Yes, this family practice had seven physician providers. There was an enormous number of nurses. There was a lab and X-ray, with a massive number of technicians.

On the ceiling was a red light, the kind of rotating beacon seen on top of police cars. "What's that?" I asked.

"When that light is on, it means there are patients waiting to be seen. It's supposed to get you to work faster."

At 8 a.m., a whistle blew. Yes, a whistle, just like in the Flintstones factory. Then a parade of patients started down what can only be described as an assembly line. Patients were greeted by one person, had their insurance checked by another, had their pulse taken by another, had their blood pressure measured by another, were weighed by another, and finally put in a room by another. Never did a patient sit when going down the line. Never was a patient at a station for more than a few seconds.

Once in a room, one of the providers went in and saw the patient for less than three minutes. The provider then went to a standing workstation where he (they were all males) dictated his notes. He then invariably pushed a button on a landline telephone that speed-dialed a local pharmacy and dictated his prescription.

Another staffer walked the patient out. The patient had had, in total, less than five minutes of time with anyone.

This was not my idea of a family practice!

I had assumed I would be shadowing FP to learn the ways of seeing family practice patients. Once again, I was wrong.

FP walked me up to a standing workstation and punched the pharmacy button. He then introduced me to the pharmacist as a new doctor in the office and instructed the pharmacist to fill all my prescriptions. This was to include controlled substances.

I was a medical student. I did not have a license to practice medicine. I most certainly could not write a prescription for anything, much less controlled substances, without being cosigned by a licensed physician. But FP then turned to me and said, "Start seeing patients."

He made it clear I was not to bother any of the doctors with questions. I was free labor, and I'd better get to work.

Well, I tried. The extent of my experience was being a third-year student. I was in over my head. I was extremely uncomfortable calling in prescriptions. But I deluded myself into thinking my charts and prescriptions would be cosigned at some point.

On my third day, the doctors had a staff meeting, to which I was invited. Finally, I hoped, there would be some discussion of medical practices and procedures. I imagined I was going to get some instruction. Wrong again.

The entire meeting involved discussing a new shopping mall the practice intended to build. There was a review of the properties the practice already owned in town (seemingly most of it). There was discussion of making sure no patient ever left the practice without a prescription, because the practice owned the pharmacy.

I was invited to FP's home that night for dinner. FP had a mansion. It was more like a castle. It was a monument to gaudy bad taste. I was treated by him and his family as a vassal who was there to fawn over FP. FP even took me outside and showed me his newly acquired motor home, all the time informing me how much every item I saw cost. He said, "You can do this if you're willing to work for it."

The next day I called the practice and said I had a meeting at the medical school. I went to the director of family practice and told her what I was doing and that I was extremely uncomfortable practicing medicine without a license.

She told me I was not to go back there.

I was relieved.

She then assigned me to a different family physician who had a solo practice in a suburb of the city.

What a difference! This man cared for his patients. He took time with them. He certainly did not make the kind of money FP made, but he was very happy.

During my time with him I was exposed to a side of medicine I had never heard of or imagined. This doctor welcomed transgender people into his practice and helped them transition, providing prescriptions for hormones and arranging for therapy of all kinds for them.

He was also the occupational medicine physician for the employees at a slaughterhouse and meat packing plant in town. He took me there one day—truly amazing! Believe me when I tell you there is no part of a cow or pig that is not used—no part at all!

This doctor also invited me to dinner one evening. His house was a standard home in a nice neighborhood. It was not ostentatious in any way. He and his family could not have been more unlike FP.

He also talked with me about single-practice finances one day. He told me how much he paid for office rent, utilities, equipment and supplies, his nurse, his receptionist/office manager, practice insurance and malpractice insurance. He then showed me the statistics on his number of visits per month and the average billing per visit. Next, he showed me the number of patients who had insurance and the percentage of his billing that insurance paid (much less). He showed me how many patients were self-pay and how many patients could not pay anything at all. He then said, "After all of that, this is what I can afford to pay myself." The amount was not great. He could have made more money in a lot of other professions.

This man taught me about family practice and I still, to this day, remember him and the lessons he so generously imparted.

Junior Internship

At the end of my third-year medical school surgery rotation, the nurses gave me an engraved pewter mug that said, "Most Promising Student in the Field of Surgery."

The nurses had never given a mug to any other student—I was the first. And I was such an ass that, when they gave it to me, I told them I was not going into surgery. I was going to be a family physician. The nurses knew better.

After my entire third year and all the mandatory rotations—medicine, surgery, pediatrics, OB/Gyn, and psych—we had to think about what we were going to take during our fourth and final year of medical school.

The fourth year consisted of clinical electives and a junior internship, or JI. During a JI, we were assigned to a single service in one of the many hospitals affiliated with the med school. We were treated as if we were doctors who had finished med school and were in our internship year.

Of course, we weren't doctors. So, although we had our own patients, wrote our own orders, made our own rounds, and even had one of two third-year students assigned to us, the nurses knew we were JIs and wouldn't take off our orders.

So, here's how things would go: the ER would page the service that was on call. If it was the JI's turn to take call for the service, the JI headed to the ER. After seeing the patient, if the JI decided to admit, the JI would write the admission orders. But no nurse was stupid enough to take off the orders or follow them.

So, the JI would do the nursing job, take off the orders, and then carry out the orders. The JI would take patients to the ward and put them in bed. The JI would send the medication orders to the pharmacy. When the meds were sent to the ward, the JI would administer the meds. The JI was doctor and nurse to the patient until the JI could get a "real" doctor (intern or resident) to cosign his orders. Once the RD (real doctor) cosigned the orders, the nurses would follow them.

Virtually everyone in my med school class took their JI in internal medicine. A handful took their JIs in pediatrics. I was the only student who elected to do a JI in surgery. In fact, the school could not remember the last time a student had taken a JI in surgery. So, they got creative and sent me to the VA Hospital that was affiliated with the med school.

I was assigned to a surgery service that had Alex as chief resident. Alex was a seventh-year resident in the seven-year residency. The sixth-year resident was Ed, who had taken me through my first ever surgery in my third year. There were three interns: me as a JI, and four third-year med students—one third-year for each of the interns and me.

It must be noted that everywhere in the country a general surgery residency was five years. Where I trained was the only seven-year program. But the director of surgery, who I will call Big WA, had an incredible ego and felt he had seven years of knowledge to pass on. In his favor, and in the residency's favor, when someone finished the seven years, they were board eligible in both general surgery and thoracic surgery. Usually when people finished a five-year surgery residency, they were board eligible in general surgery only. Then, if they wanted to do thoracic surgery, they took a two-year fellowship in that subspecialty. Alex and Ed were, in fact, fully trained general surgeons as seventh- and sixth-year residents.

Here's the scoop on Big WA. He was world-famous as the first person to treat bacterial osteomyelitis (infection of the bone) with penicillin. He did this when he was a resident, at a time when the standard of care for osteomyelitis was amputation. Big WA had a lecture that he gave about him risking his career to treat a child with osteo using penicillin. It was quite the heroic story as told by Big WA. Consequently, Big WA was a major backer of using penicillin for every possible infection.

Unfortunately, some bacteria were developing resistance to penicillin. Penicillin is a bacteriocidal antibiotic. It kills bacteria when they are dividing. Big WA allowed that, as some bacteria were becoming pen-resistant, he would allow the use of a second antibiotic in patients whose infections were not sensitive to penicillin. The second antibiotic Big WA allowed was tetracycline.

Tetracycline is a bacteriostatic antibiotic. It kills bacteria by keeping them from making normal proteins, so the bacteria cannot grow and divide.

Big WA wanted patients with resistant infections to be treated with Pen and Tet—penicillin and tetracycline. But penicillin only works when bacteria are dividing and tetracycline keeps bacteria from dividing. The literature was clear: bacteriostatic and bacteriocidal antibiotics should not be given together.

That said, Big WA was adamant. If a patient had a surgical infection, that patient was to get pen and tet. And nothing but pen and tet. If Big WA discovered one of his residents was using any antibiotic other than pen and tet that resident was fired. Firing a resident from residency was the end of their career. The now-former resident was not board eligible, could not take their board exam, and could never practice. No other program would ever consider taking on a resident who had been fired from a different program.

So, consider the plight of Alex and Ed. They were in the seventh and sixth years of residency. Had they gone anywhere else in the country they would have already graduated, taken their boards, and would be practicing surgeons. To get fired now would be disastrous.

What does all of this have to do with being at the Veterans Administration Hospital (VAH)? Things were pretty much completely run by the chief resident at the VAH. Alex got to do what he wanted because Big WA only came to the VAH for one hour on Friday mornings.

At the time of my JI at the VAH the patients were generally all WWII and Korean War veterans. We had a few WWI vets, and believe it or not, we had three Civil War vets who were all over 100 years old. All of these vets smoked. All of them had a litany of medical problems to go with their litany of surgical problems. Caring for these vets was hugely challenging.

Almost all these vets had infections to go along with their surgical problems.

Alex and Ed prescribed whatever antibiotics were indicated and appropriate. None of the patients got pen and tet.

That is, until Friday morning at 10:00 a.m.

Every Friday, the team would make our usual work rounds at 6:00 a.m. At the end of rounds, around 7:00 a.m., Alex would turn to me, the JI, and say, "Tony, you know what to do." And I would do it.

I then instructed the four third-year med students to get all the patients who were on antibiotics and physically roll their beds to the elevator and deposit them on a different floor of the VA hospital.

This usually took until around 9:00 a.m. Then we would work like fiends for an hour getting our usual amount of work done, running between our floor and the floors where we had deposited the infected patients.

At 10:00 sharp, Big WA would walk onto our ward. Big WA would only communicate with the chief resident. No one else was allowed to speak to Big WA. Big WA would look at Alex and say, "Alex, are there any patients with infections on this ward?"

Alex would say, "No sir, not a one."

Big WA would say, "If there were any infections, what would you treat them with?"

Alex would say, "Pen and tet, sir."

Big WA would then expound on the amazing quality of his surgical training, as there were never any infections on the wards when he made his rounds. We all nodded knowingly, projecting our true belief in the magic of pen and tet.

At 11:00 a.m., Big WA would depart, secure in the knowledge he was training the best residents in the country, and possibly the world, as his residents' patients never had any surgical infections.

And then the third-year students and I would go get our patients, bring them back to the ward, and treat them appropriately until next Friday's troop movement.

One of our patients on the VA service had Boerhaave's syndrome. Boerhaave's syndrome is spontaneous rupture of the esophagus. This man's ruptured esophagus had formed a tract that penetrated through his chest wall. We were keeping him on the ward and allowing the tract to slowly close spontaneously. The patient had so many medical problems, and his lungs were so damaged from years of smoking, he would have been an unsuitable surgical candidate.

One day, Alex asked me to get a barium swallow on the patient so we could see how the tract's healing was progressing. The barium would outline the esophagus, the tract coming from the side of the esophagus, and the stomach.

I got the study and got bad news. When we went down to radiology to see our films that day, we saw a large mass in what was left of the tract. The tract had closed at the skin and was closed several centimeters from the chest wall medially, but there were still six or seven centimeters of tract open from the esophagus extending into the chest cavity. In the remaining tract was a mass that appeared to be about one centimeter high and about three centimeters in length.

We were concerned that the tract had developed a cancerous tumor.

So, Alex got an endoscope and looked down the patient's esophagus and into the tract.

And saw a green bean.

The patient was supposed to be exclusively on a liquid diet while the tract healed. That meant weeks of no solid food. When we asked the patient how the green bean had gotten into his tract, he said, "I got hungry just drinking that stuff you give me, Doc. So, I been stealing food from the other patients' trays when they're asleep. Guess I got a green bean stuck down there, huh?"

Alex pulled the green bean out with the scope.

This was one of the patients we could present to Big WA on Fridays, as the patient was not infected and did not need antibiotics.

"Good judgment comes from experience. Experience comes from bad judgment." Who said that? It's been attributed to Mark Twain, Will Rogers, and Dr. Kerr L. White, according to Google. Regardless of attribution, I am the embodiment of that aphorism.

One Junior Internship afternoon, at about 4:00 p.m., I was looking up stuff in the library of the VA Hospital because I knew about a gnat's whisker more than the third-year students I was supposed to be supervising. Sitting at a table next to a window of the fourth-floor library, I saw something large fall past the window out of the corner of my eye's peripheral vision.

Peripheral vision is no better than 20/100. That means that what a person with perfect vision can see clearly from 100 feet away, your peripheral vision would have to be twenty feet away to see clearly. Peripheral vision is there, although it is blurry, to let you know something is coming and you need to turn toward it so that you can see it with 20/20 central vision.

So, I wasn't sure what had fallen, just that it was big.

I got up, looked out the window, and saw a person. That person was on top of the roof of the hospital's entrance portico. The portico roof was at a level about halfway between the second and third floors. So that person, lying unconscious, was about one-and-a-half floors below me.

What should I do? Call for help? Call a code? I had no idea. Clearly this was a patient, probably one from the psych floor up on seven, who had opened a window and jumped. But he didn't make it to the ground. He landed on the roof of the portico.

What I did was open the fourth-floor window and jump out, falling one-and-a-half stories to land next to the patient.

Did I think I could resuscitate him with the items in the pockets of my white coat? Admittedly, I had a lot of stuff in my pockets, but clearly not enough to help the guy.

When I checked him, he had a pulse and was breathing, but was unconscious. Beyond that, I had no plan.

Fortunately, someone in the library witnessed me open the window and jump out. So, when I looked up, I saw several people looking out from the fourth floor. I shouted to them to get me some help.

What help? I had no idea.

Soon the fire department arrived with a ladder truck. Firefighters raised the ladder, extracted the patient, and took him to the ER. I climbed down the ladder.

For some reason, no one congratulated me on a job well done.

For some reason, people just asked me what I was thinking when I jumped out the window.

For some reason, I didn't have a good answer.

Other than that I had used bad judgment and gained experience.

Freshman Mixer

Was I always going to be a surgeon? That was not my plan. I always intended to be a family physician in a small town.

Typing that now, I realize just how naïve it sounds—and how naïve I was.

I was the youngest person in my med school class because I had finished both high school and college in three years each. I was too immature to be in med school.

That said, when my classmates and I reported to the school for our freshman year, we were greeted by an entire week of orientation.

On the last day of orientation there was a mandatory mixer. During the mixer Dr. P, one of the deans, circulated around the room and spoke to each of us for a few minutes.

At the end of this mandatory fun, Dr. P stood on a table and called us to attention.

"I am now going to call your names, in alphabetical order, and tell you what specialty you will go into."

What? Why would he do that? We all already knew what we intended to specialize in. For the entire week we had gotten to know each other and had always asked each other, "What are you going to specialize in?"

But we hadn't considered the ego of Dr. P. He prided himself on his ability to predict our futures after speaking to us for a few moments.

One by one Dr. P called our names and announced a specialty. Each one of my classmates listened and grinned back at Dr. P when he told them their futures.

Finally, he got to the Rs. "Rizzo, you're going to be a surgeon."

I was the only student to answer back. "No, I'm not. I'm going to be a family physician in a small town."

"You just proved my point," said Dr. P.

I didn't have the social skills or maturity of the rest of the class. Most of them disagreed with what Dr. P prognosticated for them. They just had the wherewithal to keep their mouths shut. I aggressively told the dean he was wrong in front of my entire class and most of our professors.

Aggressive? Not the best social skills? Yep, sounds like a surgeon.

You're Never Going to Make It

As I write this, I am a full-time professor of anatomy and physiology. Our college goes to great lengths to nurture—or maybe, coddle—our students.

Here are a couple of examples of the kind of "nurturing" we received during my time in medical school:

In the second year we took an entire year of pathology. It was a *difficult* course. A sizable portion of the course was microscope work.

We were each required to bring our own microscope to the school. Microscopes were not provided. During the summer between college and medical school, I worked full-time and saved every penny to buy a microscope. It cost $1,000, which in 2025 money is equivalent to $7,650.69 (according to Google). I still have that microscope. From time to time my wife will ask me, "What is in that wooden box?" It's my microscope. I haven't opened the box, much less used the microscope, for decades. But I'll never part with the thing.

When my lab partner Penny dropped her microscope on her foot, every one of us asked whether-or-not she had broken her microscope. It never dawned on us to first ask about her foot.

On the day of the pathology final, it was snowing, and my car had broken down. I was in a terrible hurry to leave my apartment for one reason or another and was dependent upon hitching a ride from someone.

When my ride arrived, I rushed out, completely forgetting to bring my microscope. I didn't realize my mistake until he dropped me off at the school.

I had no way to get back to the apartment, which was over thirty minutes away, especially because the rule was if you were late to the exam, you would not be admitted, and you would fail.

I went into the building and straight to the pathology chairman's office. I explained what had happened, threw myself on his mercy, and asked to borrow a microscope. He made it very clear that I was an idiot who was not worth salvaging but begrudgingly loaned me a microscope.

A few days later, on the last day of the quarter and the day before our third-year rotations were to start, I received a message to report to the pathology chairman's office.

His secretary instructed me to stand in the hallway outside the chairman's closed door.

Standing there, I heard unintelligible shouting from inside the office. This went on for what seemed an eternity. Then the door flew open and one of my classmates rushed out past me, weeping.

This did not bode well.

I entered the office and was instructed to stand across the desk from the chairman, who was also standing.

"Rizzo, you are an idiot! You did not remember to bring your microscope to the final! You are probably the worst student I have ever seen! You passed pathology by the skin of your teeth, but I don't know how! So, you will start your rotations tomorrow! But I recommend you quit medical school right this minute because you don't have what it takes, and you will never make it!!"

My emotions were extremely mixed at that moment. I was happy and relieved I had passed pathology. I was happy I would be starting my clinical rotations the next day. But I was being shouted at by an experienced professor and physician telling me I would never make it. So, I did the only thing I could think of at the time. I asked, "May I go now?"

"Get out of my office!!"

"Yes, Sir."

My first three-month rotation on internal medicine started the next day. One morning, after being up all the previous day and night, I was sitting with my team in a small hospital conference room for sit-down rounds with the attending.

Sitting down is not advised when you have been up for more than twenty-four hours. I fell asleep.

When I awoke, much later, there was an eight-and-a-half by eleven-inch piece of paper on my lap. Scrawled on it was the message, "See me in my office" and the name of the attending.

I went to his office. He spent well over fifteen minutes berating me for falling asleep during rounds. His message, repeated many, many times, was that I did not have what it takes to be a physician and I should resign from medical school that day.

I didn't quit. Amazingly, I made it.

About my classmate who ran, crying, from the pathology chairman's office:

He was a brilliant young man. He was the only person in our class who had gotten into medical school without finishing college. It was then, and is now, the case that one can apply to medical school after completing the required prerequisites. Actually, having a bachelor's degree is not one of the prerequisites. However, with very rare exceptions, everyone who goes to medical school has completed a bachelor's degree.

This guy, TR, was so smart he was admitted to medical school after three years of college. So, he did not have an undergraduate degree.

Once in school he was excelling, as expected, when he got himself elected to national office in what was then called the American Medical Student Association. Because of his responsibilities in AMSA, he traveled around the country quite often, forcing him to miss classes.

The consequence of missing classes was he failed two classes during the second year. Normally, he would just be out. But the school took pity on him and made a major exception, allowing him to repeat the entire second year—even the classes he had passed.

He was like a haunted man during the repeat year. The pressure on him was incredible. But he failed pathology a second time. He was out.

He was also the recipient of a Health Professions Scholarship from the U.S. Air Force. The Air Force was paying his tuition, fees, books, and a salary to go to medical school. In return, the Air Force expected two years of service for the first year of the scholarship and one year for each subsequent year.

TR had received the scholarship at the beginning of the first time he was enrolled in the second year. So, he owed the Air Force three years of payback service for the two years he was supported.

But TR did not have a bachelor's degree. So, he could not enter the Air Force as an officer.

No one ever heard from TR again. Did he go into the Air Force as an enlisted man? Did he find a way to pay back the money the Air Force had invested in him?

Years later, I searched the Air Force records to try to find him. There was no record of him ever having served.

He just disappeared.

Residency

Cardiac Resuscitation War

Surgery residency involved five years of learning on the job. We learned surgery, of course, but we also learned to function in the hospital bureaucracy.

We surgery residents were caught in the middle of an actual war between the director of surgery and the director of internal medicine.

The Director of Surgery, Big Al, had written multiple papers about cardiac resuscitation. Big Al was a firm believer that closed chest CPR was worthless in resuscitation. Big Al insisted that the only way to resuscitate someone was to open their chest and perform internal cardiac massage. He literally wanted the chest to be cut open and the resuscitator's hand to be squeezing the ventricles of the heart.

The director of internal medicine was a staunch believer in closed chest CPR and thought that opening the chest was barbaric.

But we were surgery residents. And if we wanted to keep our jobs, we had to do what Big Al wanted us to do.

To understand the significance of this war between medicine and surgery, you must understand something about surgery residencies. There were two types of surgery residencies: pyramids and straight up. Our five-year surgery residency was a pyramid.

In a straight up residency, the program hired the number of interns that matched the number of chief residents it graduated. For example, my internship, taken in a different program several years prior to the rest of my residency, hired two interns each year and graduated two chief residents. **Side note:** no, I wasn't fired. I did some federal service between my internship year and my residency.] The risk of a straight up program was, if the program decided it didn't want to keep a resident for any reason—or if a resident quit—the program was ultimately short a chief resident. The American College of Surgeons and the American Board of Surgery look askance at programs that do not graduate the number of chief residents allocated to them.

One also must know that to be eligible to take the board exam in General Surgery, a resident must complete a five-year residency, do their fourth and fifth years in the same place, and be a chief resident during the fifth year. Chief resident responsibilities include running a surgery service for the entire year, under the supervision of the attendings and the director of surgery.

Thus, my internship hospital, a straight up program, had two affiliated hospitals and could graduate two chief residents. They started two interns each year and hoped they chose well.

My residency was a pyramid. We had six affiliated hospitals and graduated six chief residents. But we started with forty-two interns. What happened between the internship year and the chief year to whittle forty-two people down to six?

Most of our interns never intended to become general surgeons. They wanted a surgical specialty such as obstetrics/gynecology, orthopedics, urology, neurosurgery, ear, nose and throat, or others. Each of those surgical specialties required one or two years of general surgery as prerequisites to entering the specialty program. So, the majority of the forty-two interns self-eliminated from our general surgery program by leaving to train in a subspecialty.

However, by the third year we always had more than six residents who wanted to be general surgeons. That meant that between the third and fourth years, some of the remaining people had to be fired.

There were *so many* ways to get fired.

One of those ways was to fail to open a chest and perform internal cardiac massage at a code.

To make matters worse for us residents, because of the war between Big Al and the chief of medicine, only the medical chief resident carried a code beeper. That meant that the surgery residents had to listen for an overhead page—that always came after the code beeper went off—and run to a code to get there in time to be first, and thus, the code runner.

But we were always late because the medicine chief resident had the code beeper.

Side note: cell phones had not been invented. We carried beepers. If someone wanted you, they called the hospital operator who would send a one-way radio message to your beeper. Your beeper would then beep, and the operator's voice would come out of a little speaker in the beeper announcing what number in the hospital you were to call. If it was a code, the code beeper would announce what room the code was in. Codes were also announced in the entire hospital using overhead speakers.

One day, Big Al and the director of medicine had a war conference. During this historic event, it was decided there would be two code beepers, one for the medical chief resident and one for the surgical chief resident, set to go off simultaneously when someone called a code. Additionally, Big Al found the money to put a set of chest instruments on each of the code carts in all six of our hospitals. This was a lot of carts, a lot of instruments, and a lot of money.

But the negotiations didn't stop there. Those two lofty individuals agreed that the medical chief resident was to oversee codes for the first fifteen minutes after the residents arrived at the bedside. The medical team would do closed chest CPR and use drugs to try to start the heart and resuscitate the patient. If the patient's heart was not beating after fifteen minutes, then the surgical chief resident and his/her team were to take over. That meant opening the chest and performing open-heart massage while still using cardiac drugs.

There were a few problems with this negotiated approach to resuscitation. The biggest problem was that the brain is pretty much gone after about four minutes without oxygen. So, if the medical resuscitation was unsuccessful, the surgical attempts were *always* performed on someone who was brain dead.

Brain dead is the legal and medical definition of dead.

So, we surgery residents had no chance.

But Big Al got a report from each of our six hospitals each morning elucidating the codes in the preceding twenty-four hours. He would requisition the charts for those and check to see if the chest had been opened. If not, the surgery resident who had participated in the code was fired. There was no negotiation and no appeal.

To be honest, this was a disaster. It is horrifying to open a child's chest, especially if the parents have been ushered out of the room of their dying child and are hovering right outside of the door. But I did that. It is something beyond depressing to mutilate someone's loved one by opening their chest with the full knowledge that they are already brain dead and that there is no chance whatsoever of resuscitating them.

During my residency, I opened over one thousand chests. Of those, exactly three hearts started beating again. None of the three lived. In each case the beating heart stopped as soon as I tried to close the chest, necessitating re-opening and again trying open-heart massage. Not one survived.

But this was one way we went from forty-two interns to six chief residents.

The residents faced constant tension about potentially being fired. This level of stress, added to the inhuman hours we worked, contributed in a major way to low morale and even occasional violence.

One afternoon, I was scheduled to operate with the director of the residency program—who worked for Big Al. This attending had a *severe* personality disorder. He made it abundantly clear he did not like me. He verbally, and sometimes physically, abused me in the OR. Not once when we scrubbed together did he fail to reduce at least one of the nurses to tears.

As we were changing from our street clothes into scrubs this guy said to me, "Rizzo, what are you going to do when I fire you next week?" As this was the very end of my third year of residency, getting fired would be the end of my career.

Of course, to make sure I was as vulnerable as possible to this mind game he was playing with me, he waited until I was stripped to my undershorts to let me know he was going to get rid of me.

I stopped, turned to him and said, "You'd make me the happiest man on the surface of the Earth. I would call the Air Force, and I would be gone the next day."

"You mean they wouldn't let you finish the year?"

"Why should they?" I said. "I'm here so that the Air Force can get a surgeon. If I'm not going to be a surgeon, they would pull me out and I would be working in an ER immediately."

The significance of this conversation was that I was assigned to this civilian residency by the U.S. Air Force. I was paid by the Air Force and was on active duty during the entire residency. But, and that's a big but, the residency had never told the medical center or the university that I was being paid by the USAF. Each month my residency salary was sent to the residency to be allocated to me. But the residency was keeping what would have been my civilian salary and using the money to fund a research project.

Illegal? Probably. Unethical? Most certainly.

If I were fired, the residency would have to let the medical center and university know. My erstwhile civilian salary would end. The research project would screech to a halt.

He never again said anything to me about potentially being fired.

But the mind games continued.

Tension Pneumothorax
We Lose a Good Resident

Here's another way to get fired.

One night while I was on call during my chief residency year, one of Big Al's patients got a tension pneumothorax.

A tension pneumothorax is a collapsed lung because of increasing air pressure between the lung and the chest wall. That pressure collapses the superior and inferior vena cavae—the major veins that bring blood from the body back to the heart—resulting in loss of the heart's ability to fill. If the heart cannot fill with blood, the heart cannot pump blood.

A tension pneumothorax is high on the bad list.

The treatment for a tension pneumo is to put the biggest needle you can find in the space between the first and second ribs, immediately above the second rib, on the line that runs down from the middle of the collarbone. The pressure in the chest then escapes through the needle, the lung can expand, and the blood can return to the heart through the inferior and superior vena cavae. Then there is time to put in a chest tube, which is the definitive treatment for a pneumothorax.

On the night in question, one of the third-year residents was in charge of the surgical ICU. I'll call him Fred.

Fred wanted to be a general surgeon. That meant he had to not get fired in his third year so he could be one of the six remaining to enter the fourth and fifth years. But we had way too many third years that year. Not enough of the forty-two interns had left the program to enter other surgical specialties. So, people had to be fired.

And remember, getting fired from a surgery residency in your third year was the kiss of death for your career.

You had finished four years of college, four years of medical school, and three years of a five-year surgical residency to now have nothing. You could not sit for surgical boards. You could not practice medicine anywhere because you were not fully trained. No other residency would take you as you had been fired. If, on the off chance you could find a residency program to take you, you would have to start again as an intern—something no one would be willing to do. You *did not* want to get fired from the third year.

That day Big Al had done a partial pneumonectomy on a woman with lung cancer. That meant he took out one of her lung lobes on one side. The right lung has three lobes, and the left lung has two, so taking out a lobe is something the average person tolerates reasonably well.

But, at 3:00 a.m., the bronchial stump of Big Al's patient blew out and with each breath of the ventilator she got more and more pressure in her chest. She had a tension pneumothorax and was rapidly going to die.

Our hospital complex was huge—it covered five blocks. I was five blocks away from the surgical ICU when my pager went off to call SICU stat. I called and Fred said, "Big Al's patient has a tension pneumothorax!"

I said, "Well, you know what to do. I'm on my way."

I hung up and started running the five blocks, up and down stairs, through connecting tunnels and fire doors, using every back route I knew to get to the SICU as quickly as possible.

I finally made it to the fourth floor and into the SICU. I reached the patient's bedside to see the cardiac monitor displaying a pulse rate of less than ten beats per minute. It should be between seventy and one hundred.

I turned to Fred and said, "Didn't you put in the needle?"

"No," said Fred.

"Why not?!"

"I was afraid."

"Why?!"

"Because it's Big Al's patient, and I didn't want to make a mistake."

Of course, the nurses were seeing and hearing all of this.

I grabbed a twelve-gauge needle, shoved it into the appropriate space, and a huge rush of air and blood spurted out. Immediately the patient's pulse rate went into the seventies. A nurse and I put in another chest tube—the patient already had one from the earlier surgery—and that was the end for the moment.

One of Big Al's rules was that he was not to be called in the night. Period. That rule applied to residents. That rule most certainly did not apply to nurses. The nurses were outstanding at keeping Big Al informed of everything that occurred overnight.

So, I knew that the nurses had already informed Big Al about this event.

At 6:00 a.m. the entire surgical team always gathered in the SICU to start the day. The chief resident (me), all the other residents, and all the medical students rotating on surgery gathered prior to 6:00 to await the dramatic arrival of Big Al. This was a large number of people in the nine-bed SICU. So, we were crammed in with the nurses and patients when Big Al made his appearance.

Another of Big Al's rules was that he spoke only to the chief resident. No one else was allowed to speak to him, unless it was a nurse. Nurses were allowed to speak freely.

Big Al arrived.

Big Al looked at me and said, "Rizzo, you dumb bastard, what happened here last night?"

Big Al always called me "Rizzo, you dumb bastard." He called me that in front of the nurses, residents, other attendings, patients, and families of patients. The one and only time he didn't call me dumb bastard was at our graduation dinner at the end of the residency.

"Well, Sir," I said, "the patient you did a partial pneumonectomy on yesterday got a tension pneumothorax at about 3:00 a.m. She has another chest tube and is stable right now. I booked you OR (operating room) time for 11:00 so you can revise her bronchial stump."

Then, Big Al turned to Fred. You could have heard a pin drop, as Big Al never spoke to a lowly resident other than the chief resident.

"Fred, did you put in the needle?" Of course, Big Al had been informed by the nurses that Fred had not put in the needle.

"No, Sir. Dr. Rizzo did that."

"Fred, see me after rounds."

That was the end of Fred. He was fired that day, and we never saw him again. I have no idea what he ended up doing with his life, as none of us ever heard from him again.

Tough Diagnosis

This was not my case, but it was on my surgery service while I was a resident and is just plain interesting.

An eighteen-year-old young woman presented to the ER with a collapsed lung. If there is air in the chest cavity between the lung and the wall of the chest, that is called a pneumothorax. She required a chest tube and the tube drained blood. A chest tube is a plastic tube inserted through the skin into the space between the lung and the chest wall to suck out air, blood, or pus and re-expand the collapsed lung. It usually requires several days in the hospital.

What was causing this? She denied all traumas. She had no visible scars or signs that she had been attacked or had been in an accident.

There is something called spontaneous pneumothorax, where a bleb (outpouching of the air sacs in the lung) ruptures. Spontaneous pneumothorax is more common in young, thin, tall males. This was a young, slightly heavy, short female. But because she did not fit the classic picture did not rule out spontaneous pneumothorax, and that was her discharge diagnosis. In this case the discharge diagnosis was a WAG (wild ass guess).

One month later, she presented again with a collapsed lung. She required a chest tube and another several-day stay in the hospital. Again, she drained blood from the chest tube.

One month later the same thing happened. This time the team taking care of her ended up opening her chest in the operating room to find a collection of endometrium in her pleural space (the space between the lung and chest wall). Endometrium is the lining of the uterus. It is possible, although unusual, for endometrium to escape the uterus, travel through the bloodstream, and take up residence somewhere else in the body.

In this young woman's case, a little endometrium had migrated to her pleural space and caused her to bleed into her chest cavity every month when she had her normal menstrual flow.

The word for that is catamenial hemothorax: blood in the chest cavity related to menses and endometrium.

I never saw another case of catamenial hemothorax in my entire practice. But I never forgot that one.

Thoracic Surgery

In my fourth year as a surgery resident, I was rotated to the big central city hospital and was put on a service that covered both general surgery and thoracic surgery. The only thoracic surgeon on staff was a man we'll call TS. He was foreign-trained, spoke with a thick accent, was extremely abrupt, and was very condescending to the residents.

TS never let the residents operate—we would only assist him—which is not how surgery residents learn. So the chief residents didn't want to scrub with him. Whenever he had a case, the chief residents would pass the case to a junior resident.

For that three-month period, I was the designated thoracic surgery resident—my chief resident absolutely refused to operate with TS.

***

One patient had a three-year saga, beginning in 1985, that started with a an upper respiratory infection. The case is best explained as follows:

In September, 1985, a thirty-six-year-old patient presented to her family physical. She had an upper respiratory infection—basically, a cold. Perhaps the length of time without any improvement, or the severity of the cold triggered the FP to order a chest X-ray. There was nothing in her notes to indicate why the FP ordered the procedure.

The radiologist read the X-ray as, "Negative for pneumonia and within normal limits."

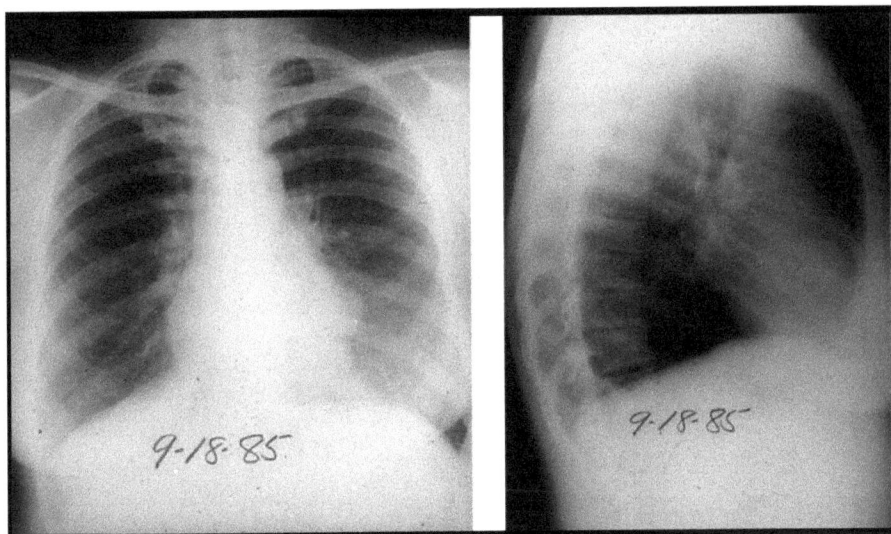

September 18, 1985 - Initial Chest Xray Posterior-Anterior and
Lateral views - negative for pneumonia

Three years later, the patient again presented to her family physician
with another cold. Again, the FP ordered a chest X-ray.

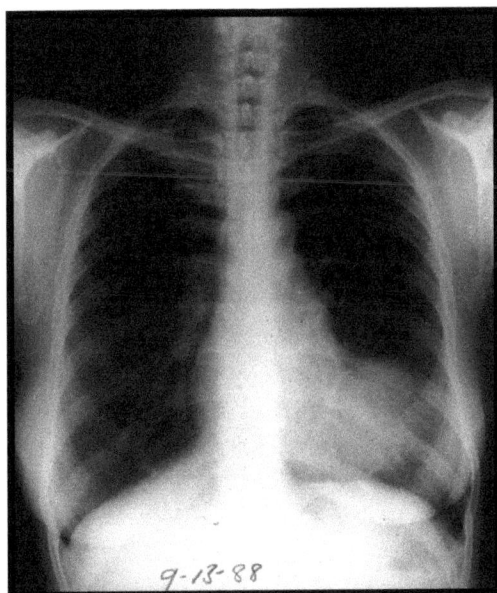

September 13, 1988 - Anterior X-ray
showing mass

These films were almost exactly three years apart. You can see a large mass in the left chest against the patient's heart. The radiologist read the mass and reported it to the family physician who never saw the films himself. He depended on reading the radiology reports as so many doctors do.

Based on the radiologist reporting a left chest mass, the family physician referred the patient to thoracic surgery. The family physician made the referral "routine" as opposed to "urgent" or "stat." Because the referral was routine, I did not see the patient in clinic until three weeks later.

I had the radiology report. After speaking with the patient and examining her, I ordered a repeat X-ray.

The difference is I always looked at my films myself. So, when I sent the patient to the X-ray department I included in the order, "Please page me as soon as the X-rays are completed."

When I got the page, I left the clinic and walked down to radiology. The mass in her left chest was clearly visible on both the PA (posterior to anterior) and lateral views.

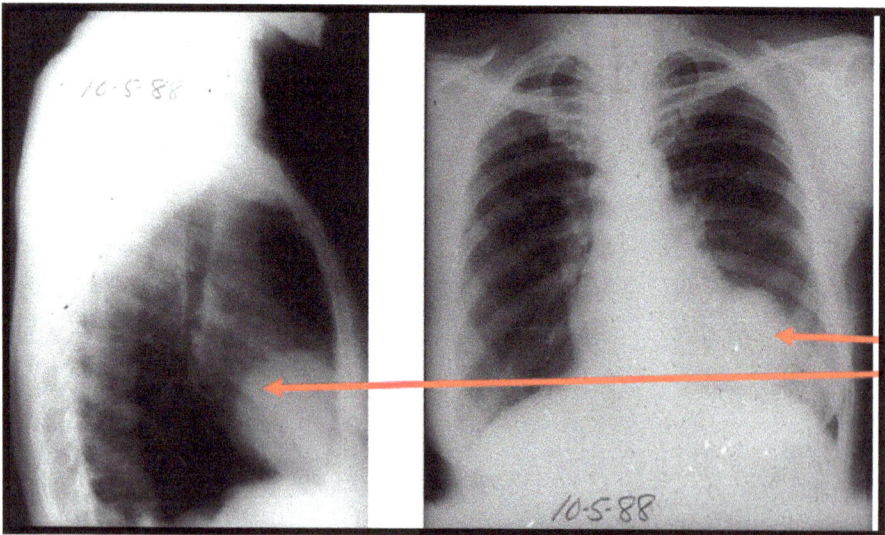

**October 5, 1988 - PA and lateral views showing the mass.
The red arrows mark the mass.**

Clearly, that mass had to have been around for a while to have grown that big. So, I had the patient's previous films pulled and looked at them. The original film from three years previous that you have already seen—the one read as "negative" by the radiologist is on the next page.

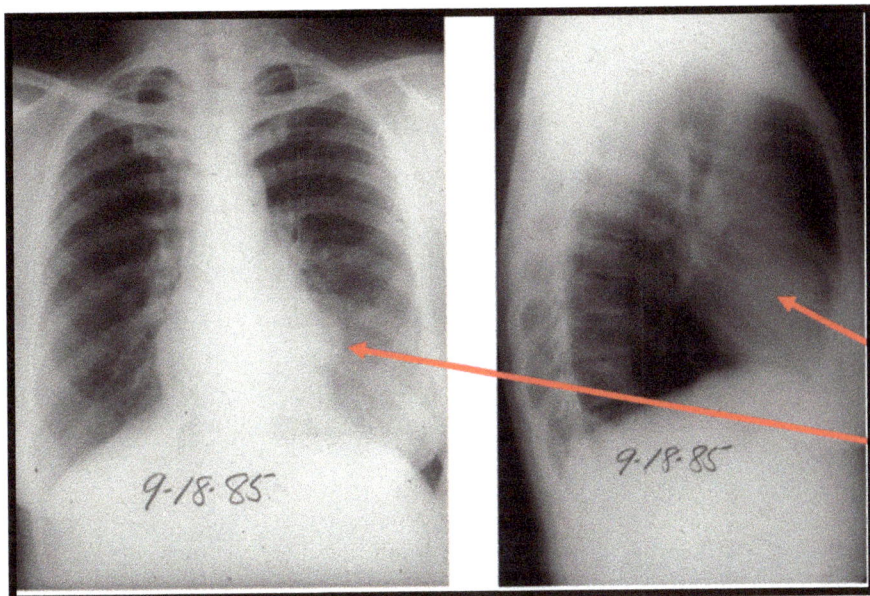

September 18, 1985 - Initial Chest Xray Posterior-Anterior and Lateral views. The red arrows marked the missed mass.

The mass is there on both the PA and lateral views. The radiologist had missed it three years before. That's because the film was read by a radiology resident and was not checked by an attending.

Since the family practice doctor did not look at his own films, this patient did not have the benefit of a second pair of eyes that might have seen the mass.

The fact that this mass had been present for more than three years told me a great deal, however. It was a big mass. Yet the patient did not have any respiratory symptoms or complaints. She had no shortness of breath and no cough. She had no weight loss. She had no change in appetite or exercise tolerance. In fact, she denied any symptoms or complaints of any kind. She had never smoked, but she had lived in a city with a high degree of air pollution for her entire life.

I reasoned if this was a cancer she most certainly would be symptomatic, and it probably would have already taken her life.

Clearly, though, this thing had to come out.

Several questions had to be answered prior to going to the OR. Was this mass attached to the heart? Did it have an extensive blood supply? Answering just those two questions would help us to plan the case. Additionally, we needed to know the patient's pulmonary functions in case we had to take out some lung.

We sent her to CT and discovered the mass was touching the heart but was not part of the heart.

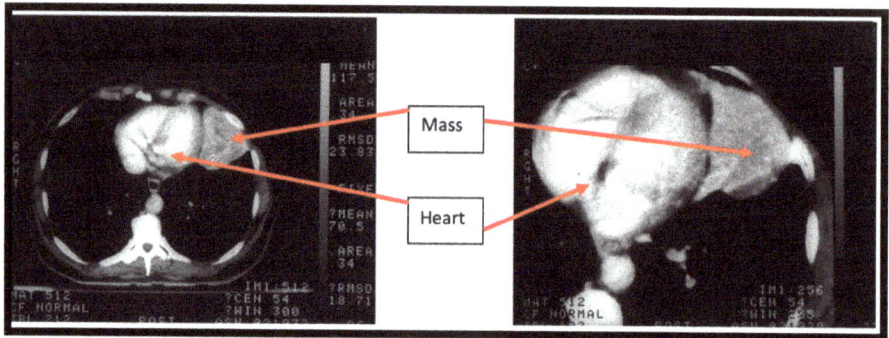

October 18, 1988 - CT of chest

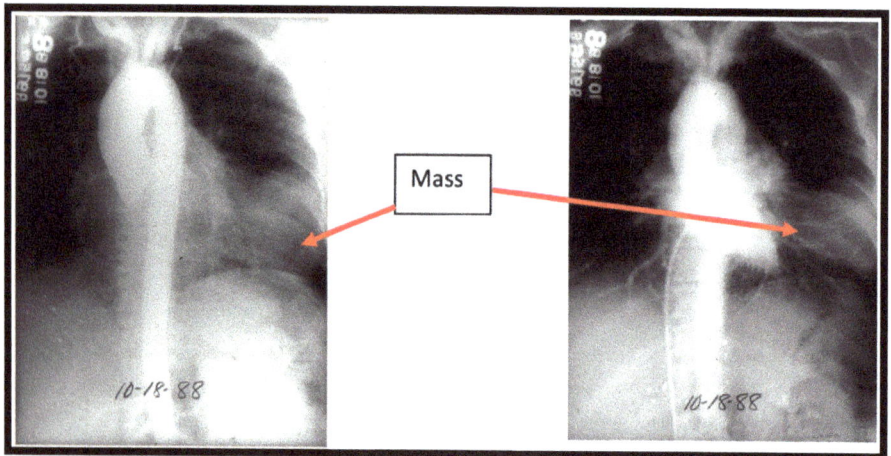

October 18, 1988 - Venogram and Arteriogram of mass

Both a venogram and an arteriogram demonstrated extensive vascularity, so we knew this had the potential to be a bloody case.

We were pretty certain this was going to be benign and not a cancer, but it was growing and pressing on the surface of the heart, so it had to come out. Even benign masses can and do cause damage by pressing on adjacent or surrounding structures.

When we got to the OR we found exactly what we expected: a highly vascular mass.

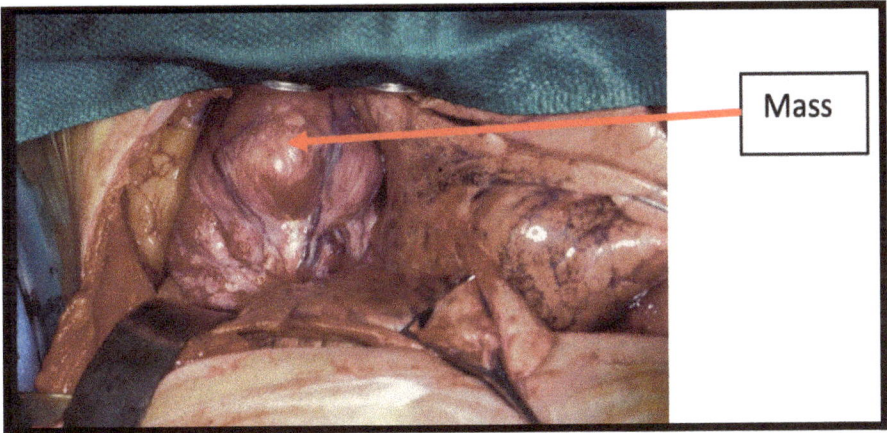

Mass sitting on heart

As it was benign it was touching, but not physically attached to the heart. Thus, it was easy to pull away from the surface of the pericardium (covering of the heart). I successfully removed the mass.

You can see that the surrounding lung is streaked with black material. As already stated, this woman never smoked, but she lived her entire life in a major city that was heavily air polluted.

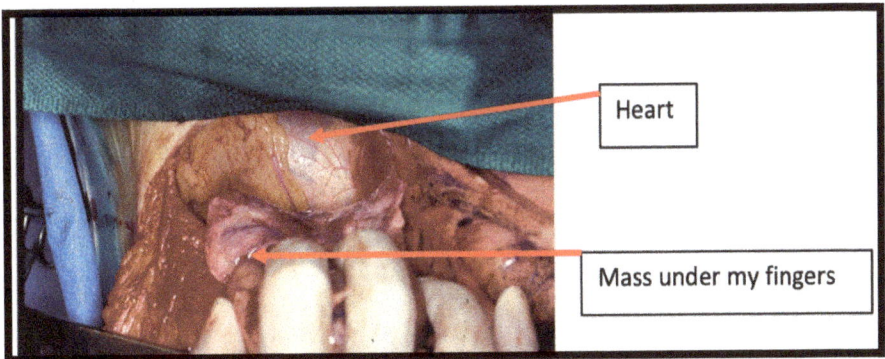

Mass peeled from heart

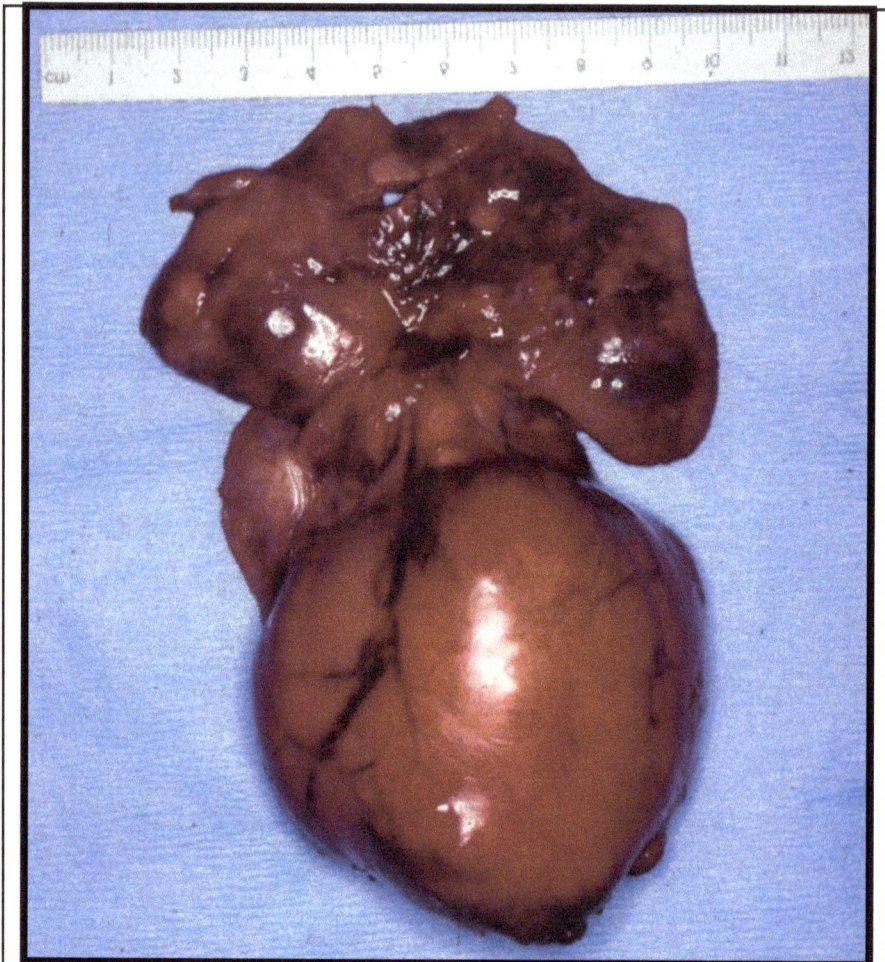

This is the mass on a back table in the OR after we removed it.

Post-operatively the patient had an uneventful recovery.

Pathology told us it was a hamartoma. A hamartoma is a benign tumor of tissue that is "normal" tissue but that develops abnormally. So, this was a benign tumor of lung in the lung.

It was a very interesting case.

Why You Have To Be NPO

Cheeseburger Pneumonia

NPO is Latin for *nolo per oris*, which translates as "nothing by mouth." Surgeons want their patients to be NPO for at least eight hours before surgery for one very good reason: vomit.

When the anesthesiologist puts someone to sleep in the operating room they intubate the patient. That means a plastic tube is inserted into the mouth, through the vocal cords, and into the trachea (breathing tube). The anesthesiologist then breathes for the patient through that tube during the case. Why? Because to put a person to sleep in the OR also means paralyzing them, and paralyzed patients cannot breathe on their own.

At the end of the case, the anesthesiologist gives drugs that reverse the paralysis and, when the patient is adequately waking from the anesthetic agent, the anesthesiologist will extubate the patient—the breathing tube is pulled out.

When the tube is pulled through their vocal cords, all patients gag. If there is something in their stomach, the patient will vomit when the vocal cords are stimulated by the tube's removal.

But the patient will still be anesthetized, although lightly—remember the patient is waking up. They are not deep enough to operate upon, but they are not totally conscious and cannot protect their own airway.

Vomiting at this rather critical moment can result in aspiration of the vomit, which means some of the vomit that was coming up through the esophagus can go right down the trachea into the lungs.

Stomach contents are acidic from stomach acid. Acidic stomach contents in the lungs results in aspiration pneumonia, a form of chemical pneumonia that has approximately a 15% mortality rate.

So, patients who are going under general anesthesia are placed NPO at least eight hours before the case—if there's nothing in your stomach, you can't vomit and aspirate.

During my residency, one of our attendings was trying to write the definitive paper on morbid obesity surgery. He would operate on anyone regardless of their underlying medical conditions, which ultimately resulted in him losing his surgical privileges because he had such a high rate of both morbidity and mortality.

We hated operating with this attending because we were the ones who had to try to keep these patients alive after surgery—he was only interested in the surgical case itself and never made rounds, nor was he invested in the patients once the case was over.

All his patients were train wrecks. They were poorly controlled diabetics, had lung diseases, had skin infections, usually smoked, and, of course, were morbidly obese. As the morbid obesity surgery was all open, meaning through large abdominal incisions—doing these cases through laparoscopes was decades in the future—they all had horrible post-op courses. He would admit them prior to the surgical date so we residents could "tune up" the patients. "Tuning up" meant trying to get the patients into some semblance of health that would be adequate to undergo the rigors of the big procedure he planned to do.

A day or two in the hospital was not adequate to reverse a lifetime of disease. Hence, we hated trying to take care of these patients who frequently did poorly, or died, postop.

Side note: Today, morbid obesity surgery is routinely performed in community hospitals via laparoscopes and is an outstanding way to help morbid obesity patients. The risks of laparoscopic morbid obesity surgery are minimal. And—this is wonderful—90% of today's recipients of morbid obesity surgery who have type 2 diabetes are diabetes-free one year after their surgery. But this was all in the future when I was a resident.

One of this attending's admissions was a 400-pound woman whom he admitted the day before surgery. We had no chance of "tuning her up." We did what we could, wrote the NPO order for midnight before the day of surgery, and took her to the OR at 8:00 a.m. the next morning.

When the anesthesiologist extubated her, she vomited and aspirated. Now this immense woman, who had a huge abdominal incision and had undergone a massive surgical case, also had aspiration chemical pneumonia. She would require weeks of intensive care.

Her time in the hospital was horribly complicated and could fill a book all by itself. I will only tell you this: one day, when we were getting the better of her many, many complications and she was able to speak, I asked her about how it became possible for her to have vomited a rather massive amount of emesis. I knew I had explained to her why she had to be NPO, and I had written the order. The nurses had made sure there was nothing to eat in her room.

"Well, doctor, after the nurses took all of the food from my room at midnight the night before surgery, I got pretty hungry. So, I snuck out of my room, eloped from the ward, and took the elevator down to the cafeteria. I got six cheeseburgers from the vending machine, ate them really fast, and snuck back before any of the nurses knew I was gone."

That explained the vomit.

It also allowed me to report what may be the only case on record of "cheeseburger pneumonia."

Something Moving

There were several years between my surgical internship and residency while I did some federal service—another story for another time. I found out I was going to perform that service approximately halfway through my internship year. That's because the Feds had paid for my medical school with a Health Professions Scholarship. I had been promised I would not have to perform the federal service payback years until after my residency was completed.

Nope. We want you as soon as you finish your internship year, they decided.

I went to the director of the residency and told him I would not be able to complete the residency, as he and I had understood, when he accepted me into this "straight up" program. He was a gracious gentleman and took the news in stride. I then asked him if I could modify the remaining six months of the internship year by spending some time on internal medicine and obstetrics.

He agreed. Soon after that he paid me one of the highest compliments he could when he asked me, an intern, to repair a laceration on his teenage daughter's face.

I delivered 300 babies during one month on obstetrics. It was every other night of call. I solidified my belief that you must be someone special to make obstetrics your life's work.

On internal medicine, I was truly a fifth wheel, but the medicine attending and residents tolerated me and taught me a lot.

"Do you have any questions?" the medicine attending asked one morning at the end of rounds. Neither of the medicine residents did. I spoke up. "When we give nitroglycerine for chest pain, why don't the patients blow up?"

The attending physician and the residents stared at me for a long while. The attending then silently turned and walked away.

Hey, I thought that was funny! They didn't.

My last month of internship, in May, was on anesthesia.

I was immediately thrown into the OR to give anesthesia to surgical patients under the direct supervision of a board-certified anesthesiologist attending.

I did three cases that first day. I intubated the first two patients and put them on the vent for my surgical colleagues. The last case of that first day was a beautiful, blond-haired, five-year-old girl. She was going to have a minor case that would take less than ten minutes of anesthesia time. Because the case was going to be so short, the anesthesia attending told me to just hold a mask over the patient's nose and mouth and breathe for her using a bag. That way the patient would not have a sore throat when we woke her up.

But it also meant I had to have perfect technique to keep the mask sealed by holding it with one hand while breathing for the patient by squeezing the bag with my other hand.

"How are you doing, Rizzo?" asked the anesthesia attending.

"Fine."

Out of the blue, the attending then said, "Hooray, hooray! The first of May! Outdoor sex begins today!"

Not what I expected from an attending, especially one I felt was ancient (she was probably in her fifties).

Then she said, "Rizzo, did you notice the patient's eyebrows are moving?"

No, I had not noticed that. But now I did.

This beautiful little angel of a girl had head lice actively crawling around her eyebrows. And her hair. And her head was essentially in my lap as I sat at the head of the table unable to move away because I had to hold the mask and bag her.

After the case was done, I went down to the hospital laundry, disposed of my scrubs, and took a shower with some Permethrin (lice killer) I got from the pharmacy.

I never saw any lice on me, but I itched for several days.

Chief Residency

Chief Residency - Introduction

Performing surgery is an awesome responsibility. People trust you to render them unconscious, then inflict upon them what would be a fatal wound if it occurred outside of the operating room, then muck about through their insides, frequently leaving them with fewer organs than what they started with.

So, to learn what needs to be learned, surgery training is long. Surgery training is rigorous. Surgery training is relentlessly self-critical.

During the chief residency year, the fifth-year resident is expected to run a surgery service. As my program graduated six chief residents each year, we had six major hospitals as part of the program. Each chief resident would spend three months at a time at a hospital running all the surgery services and residents. That meant acting as an attending physician when on call and making the schedules for everyone and everything.

Of course, the chief resident was still a resident, so he or she should have been able to call an attending physician whenever needed. In my program, the chief residents were expected to make such a call rarely. That said, whether-or-not one called the attending depended upon which hospital one was in at the time.

At one of the hospitals in the center of the city, where the patients were primarily indigent and persons of color, the attendings did not want to be called—ever. Racist? Very much so!

At one of the suburban hospitals, where the patients usually had insurance and were Caucasian, the attendings demanded to be called for pretty much everything. Racist? You bet!

Chief residents had to learn to be flexible.

But back to surgery training being relentless and self-critical.

M & M
(Morbidity & Mortality)

Every Saturday morning the entire surgery program would assemble—unless you were working in the OR or ER—for M & M conference. For each of the six surgery services the chief resident stood in front of the assembled masses and presented every complication (morbidity) and every death (mortality) on the service for the previous week.

The assembled masses were all the attendings from all the hospitals as well as community surgeons, most of whom we had never met. After the chief resident presented each case, the attendings were encouraged to ask questions. By "ask questions" what is meant is verbally attack the chief resident and the residents who had anything to do with the care of the patient.

It was brutal.

From time to time, a junior resident was asked to present at M & M. The attendings' usual goal was to reduce that resident to tears. If they succeeded in making a chief resident cry, he could expect to be fired that day.

Two cases I had to present—a couple weeks apart—involved the same intern. Unfortunately, both were mortalities. After I presented the second case, we never saw that intern again. We didn't know if he was fired or if he resigned.

Both deaths were tragic.

The intern was a brilliant man who should have had an excellent career ahead of him. Losing him was also tragic.

The first case was that of an infant in the pediatric intensive care unit (PICU) who was being covered by my service for a non-operative surgical problem. There are many surgical problems that are not operated upon, and this was one of them. The baby was far from out of the woods but was slowly improving and expected to make a full recovery and go home to his loving family.

Back to the racism aspect: this was a case in a suburban hospital and the family was Caucasian. So, the attending was interested in the case since he got paid for being involved in it.

One night on call, at about 3:00 a.m, one of the PICU nurses called the intern to say labs had come back on the baby, and the baby's serum potassium was low. It is important to keep all patients' blood electrolytes in balance so they can heal from their diseases or wounds. Low potassium is dangerous for anyone, especially babies.

But—and this is a big but—a high serum potassium is also dangerous. Too high and the heart can stop.

So, the intern went up to the PICU, looked at the chart, saw the baby's weight and his potassium level, and calculated a dose of potassium to try to correct the low value. He wrote an order for the calculated dose and left the PICU to continue the immense amount of work a surgical intern had to do all night, every night.

The nurse took the order off and sent it to the pharmacy. The nurse should have also done the dosage calculation to confirm the intern's math was correct. She was busy, the intern was known to be very smart, and it was 3:00 a.m., so she didn't do her own math. She trusted the doctor.

Pharmacy got the order, filled it, and sent the potassium for IV administration up to PICU. The pharmacist should have done the dosage calculation to confirm the doctor's order. But the pharmacy was busy, the pharmacist assumed that the nurse had confirmed the intern's math, and it was 3:00 a.m., so the pharmacist sent the medication up to PICU without checking.

When the potassium arrived in PICU the nurse should have done a calculation to confirm the dosage was correct. But she was busy and assumed that the pharmacist had done his check, so she just gave the IV potassium.

Unfortunately, the intern had made a math error. He misplaced a decimal point and wrote a dose ten times more than the baby needed.

The massive amount of potassium stopped the baby's heart.

I heard "Code Blue, PICU" announced overhead and on my code beeper.

I, and the rest of the team, coded the baby for a long time to no avail. This baby should have gotten well and gone home. Instead, the infant was dead due to the intern's math error and failure of the nurse and the pharmacy to do their jobs.

The only reason the intern was not fired on the morning I presented the case to M & M was because the nurse and pharmacist were accessories.

But the error was the intern's.

To say the critique was brutal does not begin to describe it, especially from the attending on the case.

A couple weeks later, I again presented a death at M & M involving the same intern.

This death was in a sixteen-year-old female in the same suburban hospital. Her family was wealthy and Caucasian. The attending was interested in the case. Racist? Perhaps. Economic? Likely.

This girl was in renal failure and on the transplant list. She was admitted to my service for an infection. Normally an infection would have gone to medicine, but, because she was on the transplant list, any-and-all medical problems she might have were to be managed by surgery.

While she was in the hospital, she was going down to dialysis every three days.

One dialysis day, a nurse called the intern at 4:00 p.m. because she saw that the patient's serum potassium was low. Between 6 a.m. and 4 p.m. the patient had gone to dialysis, but the nurse had received the lab result at 6:00 a.m.

It is unknown why the nurse did not tell the intern that the patient's low potassium study was from ten hours earlier and obtained prior to dialysis. The intern did not ask when the low potassium lab had been obtained. He simply heard the nurse report a low serum potassium and responded by ordering a standard dose of IV potassium appropriate for the patient's age and weight.

Why did the intern not ask when the potassium had been drawn? Probably because the intern had been up all the previous day, all the previous night, and now it was 4:00 p.m. He was exhausted—the typical state of being for residents.

The nurse sent the order to the pharmacy. Pharmacy sent the potassium up to the floor. The nurse gave the potassium.

The patient's heart stopped.

I heard "Code Blue, 4 West" announced overhead and on my code beeper.

Because it was about 5:00 p.m. when she coded, her family was visiting at her bedside. We sent them into the hallway where they hovered during our unsuccessful attempts to resuscitate her. We coded that girl for a long time to no avail.

And, because Big Al was the director of surgery, I opened her chest. So, we gave the family a dead daughter whose body we had mutilated after we killed her with potassium.

I spent hours preparing that M & M presentation. The reason was that I had ordered labs to be drawn during the code. The patient's serum potassium came back as 7.3mg%. Normal serum potassium is around 4mg%. A potassium of 7.3 is unheard of and incompatible with life. I had never seen a potassium level that high.

I sent a sample of the patient's IV bottle to the lab and had them calculate the amount of potassium the intern ordered. The amount was what the intern had ordered, so it was not an error on the part of the pharmacy.

I then asked dialysis what the patient's serum potassium had been when she left their unit. They said they did not know because they never normally checked.

This was both shocking and eye-opening to me. I had never been to the dialysis unit and had never had anything to do with what goes on there. That was up to the medicine people. So, I had to learn our dialysis unit's standard procedures.

It turned out that the unit never checked serum potassium, either before or after dialysis. The dialysis folks just had a standard dialysis fluid they used. So, I back calculated what the patient's serum potassium had to have been when she left the dialysis unit and before the intern ordered more potassium for her. She had, according to my calculations, a potassium of 6mg% at the end of dialysis, which is also dangerously high and usually would not be compatible with life.

I asked a nephrologist how it was possible for the patient to have a potassium of 6 and still be alive. He told me patients in renal failure for long periods of time acclimate to high potassium levels. I had never heard or read that, but I had to believe him.

So, my intern ordered potassium at 4:00 p.m. based on a lab that was ten hours old, did not know that after dialysis her potassium was not low but was horribly high, and the additional potassium he gave killed her.

Killed her in front of her family who had to be there while I opened her chest.

Try to imagine how brutal that M & M was.

That intern, a very smart guy who intended to be a general surgeon, disappeared from the program and was never seen or heard from again.

Learned by Experience

At the time I was a resident, general surgery residency was five years long. It was that lengthy because it takes time to be exposed to all the pathology and all the surgeries one might encounter once in practice. It also takes time to learn the judgment required when deciding when or if to operate.

Also, at the time I was a resident, internal medicine residency was three years long.

At night, when on call, that meant the Surgical ICU (SICU) was usually covered by a third-year surgery resident while the Medical ICU (MICU) was typically covered by either an intern or second-year resident.

The difference in experience was telling.

One evening around 6:00 pm, I got paged to go to the MICU. The nurses asked me to come down and help them put in a central IV line. A central line is put into a large, central vein such as the sub-clavian (under the collarbone or clavicle) to monitor the pressure in the central veins. A central line can also be used as an IV to give hyperalimentation, which is putting proteins, fats, and carbohydrates directly into the bloodstream when the gut cannot be used.

I went down to MICU and put in the central line for the nurses, then paused as I was walking out of the unit. Why did I pause? Because it was my habit to look in each room as I walked by. Patients, especially patients in ICUs, need as many eyes on them as possible. That's why they are in a unit. I didn't like what I saw in one of the rooms.

One of the patients was a man, approximately forty-five years old. The head of his bed was elevated to about fifty degrees. He was leaning back on the bed, clearly exhausted, and using his accessory muscles to breathe.

Humans usually breathe with their diaphragm and the intercostal muscles, the muscles between their ribs. But there are accessory muscles that can be used. Those muscles are found in the shoulders, back, and neck and raise the entire rib cage to inhale. If you have ever run a long distance (or short distance if you're out of shape), you probably used accessory muscles to inhale while you were gasping to "get your breath back."

This patient was using accessory muscles to inhale while in bed.

I waved the medical resident over who was covering the MICU that night. He was an intern.

"That guy is using his accessory muscles to breathe," I said. "He's going to exhaust himself at around midnight and will have to be intubated then and put on a ventilator. Since I'm already here, do you want to intubate him now and put him on a vent?"

"No!" the intern replied. "He's here because he's septic, not because he needs help breathing."

Of course, sepsis is the leading cause of death in ICUs in the United States. This man's sepsis was clearly trying to kill him.

"OK," I said. "He's your patient and this is your unit. But if he was in the SICU, we'd intubate."

"That's the difference between medicine and surgery," said this first-year intern to me, a fifth-year resident. "We know what we're doing."

I shrugged, looked at the nurses, and said, "OK, no problem. I'll be seeing you later."

At 11:58 p.m. my code beeper went off. "Code Blue, MICU," came over the beeper and the overhead speaker.

I ran down to the MICU. Guess who had stopped breathing? We intubated the patient, did CPR, gave drugs, and put him on a vent after getting his pulse back.

I didn't say, "I told you so." I didn't have to. Residency is about learning the art and science of the practice of medicine. I was in my fifth year of training after medical school. The MICU doctor was in his first year. He learned something that night.

Did that make me a better doctor than the MICU intern? No. It just made me more experienced.

New State Law

While I was in the middle of my chief year, something happened that had never happened either before or since: Big Al called a mandatory meeting of all the residents from all six hospitals in the middle of the day in the middle of the week. Big Al's secretary called the six chief residents, stating there were to be no excuses. Everyone was to attend.

We all trooped to the meeting, some from as far away as fifty miles, leaving patients and a ton of work to be done.

We all looked at Big Al who laconically made his announcement. "The state legislature, in its infinite wisdom, has passed a new law. From now on residents will have to work no more than sixty hours per week."

What?!

This law was written as the result of a successful lawsuit from a family who lost a loved one in a teaching hospital just like ours. The lawsuit claimed, successfully, that the family's loved one died as the result of a resident's error and that the error was the result of the resident being exhausted. The state legislature was going to fix resident exhaustion by limiting our work hours.

How would that be possible? The average work week for a surgery resident was double that—120 hours/week. Since there are 168 hours in a week, that meant that normally surgery residents worked forty straight hours, got a little sleep, then started another forty straight hours, then repeated *ad infinitum* for five years. We were all exhausted, always. One of the other chief residents had recently disappeared for several hours. We were worried when he called from upstate. He had gotten into his car and gone into a fugue state—literally driving while asleep—and ended up a couple hundred miles to the north when he woke up at the wheel, didn't know where he was, and pulled over to call us.

Given the number of hospitals and services we had to cover, it would be physically impossible to cut our hours in half and still get the job done.

Plus, what if we were in the middle of an operation when we hit the magic number? Were we supposed to leave a patient on the operating table?

"Rizzo!" said Big Al. "Make a schedule that complies with the new law and still gets all of the services covered."

I looked at the other five chief residents and they looked back at me. I had had the rose pinned on me. Clearly none of them were going to open their mouths, and the junior residents knew better than to speak to Big Al. So, I asked, "How are we supposed to get all of the services covered 24/7/365 with the number of residents we have if we cut our hours in half?"

"Rizzo, you dumb bastard, I just told you to make the schedule."

"I heard you, Sir. But it is mathematically and physically impossible to do all that we have to do and limit our residents to sixty hours per week."

Big Al was not used to anyone arguing with him, especially in front of the entire surgical residency.

"Rizzo, you dumb bastard, I gave you an order, and I expect it to be followed."

"What you are asking is impossible, Sir."

Big Al stared at me for a long, long moment. Then he said, "Make a schedule that obeys the new law, and that's what we will send to the state. Then keep making the real schedule like we always have done it."

"Understood, Sir."

The state blithely assumed our huge program covering six hospitals was obeying the law because they saw the schedule I wrote. We were still working 120-hour weeks, were still exhausted, and babies and sixteen-year-old dialysis patients were still dying as the result of errors made by exhausted residents.

Perversion

One of the hospitals I spent three months in during my chief resident year had been a significant part of my second through fifth years. Many of my rotations had been in that hospital. I knew the nurses and staff, and they knew me.

The Surgical ICU (SICU) at that hospital was on the fourteenth floor. It was nine beds and was run by an attending I'll call Dr. S.

This hospital was in the center of a major metropolis and thirty miles from our residency program's parent hospital. There were shootings and stabbings every day of the year, many of which ended up in our ER. If the victims lived, they ended up in our SICU.

Our SICU was always full. When we had more patients than could fit, we had to keep them in the ER—sometimes for days—while awaiting a SICU bed. Never was there a time when SICU had an empty bed. Never.

We almost never saw Dr. S. When we did, we dreaded it. He was not current as a surgeon. He basically never operated. He just ran the unit and did it in a very hands-off manner. When he did make rounds, he almost always asked us to do something that was surgically or medically incorrect.

We all learned to tell Dr. S we would follow his orders. Then we would wait for him to leave and ignore what he had told us to do. Since he never followed up, he was none the wiser. And the patients got better.

That all changed one afternoon, about 6:00 pm. Dr. S appeared in the unit and had the third-year resident page me. I went up to fourteen to be told, "Rizzo, I have a patient I want to move from the floor to the SICU. Make a bed."

What that should have meant was that another surgery attending had called Dr. S, said he had a patient on a ward that needed ICU care, and asked Dr. S for help.

But that's not what it meant.

Dr. S was a pervert. He had an obsession for large-breasted African American women. From time to time, he would walk through the wards of the hospital looking for such a woman. When he found one, he would read her chart. If she had a surgical problem, he would introduce himself as the SICU director and tell her he wanted to personally assume responsibility for her care. Since the patients were accustomed to the standard racism of the hospital, they were almost always happy to have someone tell them he was a director and wanted to help them.

Dr. S had found such a patient. She had a relatively minor surgical problem, was recovering, and, in fact, was almost ready for discharge.

In the SICU at that time all nine beds were filled with extraordinarily complex surgical patients. All were gunshot wound victims, and none were anywhere near stable enough for transfer to a ward.

I told Dr. S that none of the current SICU patients could be moved. He became infuriated. He told me he was the attending, he was the SICU director, I was a lowly resident, and if I didn't want to be fired two months before I was due to graduate from residency, I would do exactly what he wanted me to do.

Dr. S would, indeed, have called Big Al and told him to fire me. Big Al would have done it.

But none of the current ICU patients could be moved from the intensive care they needed.

And, if left alone, Dr. S would molest the woman he wanted moved to the SICU.

I needed a plan, and this is what I came up with: first, I went to see the woman. Indeed, she was ready for discharge in a couple of days and certainly did not warrant a SICU bed.

Second, I went to the head nurse of the medical ICU. I had known her for my entire residency, and we had a good relationship. For fear of breaking my own arm by patting myself on the back, we had a good relationship because I was one of the few surgery residents who treated the nursing staff with respect. I told the MICU head nurse we were horribly in need of another ICU bed and asked if I could move one of my SICU patients into her unit. I promised—and she knew I would keep my promise—that one of the surgery residents would provide all the care the patient would need. I told her it would be for only a couple of days. Thankfully, she agreed.

Third, I called together all the surgery residents assigned to that hospital and told them what was happening. You can imagine how happy they were (not!). I told the residents that under no circumstances was Dr. S to be unaccompanied when he came to the SICU to see the woman we were transferring in. They all understood and agreed.

So, one of our very sick SICU gunshot-wound patients moved to MICU. The woman moved from a ward to SICU. Dr. S intermittently appeared to see her, pulled the curtains around her bed, and was immediately accompanied by a resident who was "there to help."

After two days and nights of Dr. S becoming frustrated by not ever being alone with the patient, he paged me and told me to discharge the woman. "She's fine and doesn't need ICU care," he said.

Our gunshot wound patient transferred back to SICU. The woman left the hospital without being molested. I kept my job and could graduate in two months.

But Dr. S was still the horrible person and terrible doctor that he was. The administration wanted to hear nothing about him.

I saved one woman but could not eliminate the problem that was Dr. S.

Last Day

Finally, the big day arrived—my last day of residency. I was chief resident in the same central city hospital where Dr. S ran the SICU.

I was on the fourteenth floor with the fourth-year resident who would be chief resident the next day. I had been up all night and all the previous day, and it was now 8:00 a.m.

"Trauma Code, ER" came over the beeper and was announced overhead.

Fourth Year and I looked at each other and headed for the stairs. We always ran up and down the fourteen flights of stairs, as using the elevator would take too long (I was in pretty good shape in those days).

In less time than you can imagine we arrived in the ER to find a young man of color on a gurney. The intern and third-year resident covering the surgical side of the ER were at the bedside.

The patient was shot in the kneecaps, penis and scrotum, abdomen, chest, and head. The only reason his heart was still beating, and he was still breathing, was because he was young. Anyone older would already be clinically dead.

This was a standard occurrence in our ER. Drug dealers sometimes needed to send a message to their underlings, especially underlings they suspected of ripping them off. So, they would first shoot their victim in the knees. Now he's down. Then they would shoot their reproductive organs. In this case, the bullet got both the penis and scrotum. Then they would shoot the abdomen, but usually in the left lower quadrant to not yet kill the victim. Then they would shoot the chest, usually on the right side to miss the heart and keep the victim alive for a little more torture. Finally, they would shoot the head.

But, because these drug dealers were young, they sometimes didn't die right away and would find their way to our ER. Invariably these people were brain dead from the final wound to the head, but it was a shame that we never could harvest organs from these guys for transplants. The abdominal organs had been spoiled by the abdominal gunshot wound and the heart was usually compromised by the chest wound, even though the heart had not been hit.

This man was going to take hours of time, since we were morally obligated to try to resuscitate him as he still had a heartbeat and was breathing from his one working lung. But clearly, after hours and hours of fruitless labor, we would turn off all the IVs and the ventilator when we were able to get the tests that confirmed he was brain dead.

I turned to the tomorrow-to-be-fifth-year and said, "I can't take another one of these. He's all yours."

I turned and walked out of the hospital, got in my car, and drove the forty-five miles home. I never checked out of the hospital, never turned in my badge, never said final goodbyes. I was done. Done.

I was, as Frank Burns had been described in M*A*S*H, "emotionally exhausted and morally bankrupt."

Active Duty

Introduction

"It's an honor to serve a great Nation."

Aman said that to me as he checked my receipt on the way out of Costco. He was wearing a Vietnam Veteran ball cap. I was wearing my uniform. I told him, "Welcome home," something he most likely did not hear when he came back from Vietnam.

"It's an honor to serve a great Nation," was his response.

I was honored to serve this great Nation for thirty-nine-and-a-half years. Here are a few patients who stand out in my memory...

But, first, a rant that again involves breaking my arm by patting myself on the back:

One day at the U.S. Air Force Academy Hospital, the infection control nurse came up to my office and said, "Dr. Rizzo, you are the only surgeon in any specialty to have had not a single surgical wound infection in two years. What is your secret?"

Surgical wound infections are the bane of a surgeon's—and their patients'—existence. When the infection control nurse told me that, I had not realized that I had gone two years without an infection. But I had certainly seen plenty of infections when covering for the other surgeons. Sometimes surgical wound infections required additional surgery.

So how did I manage it?

Two tactics.

First, I was gentle with the tissues. I always used instruments on the skin with great care. I did not want to crush and kill cells. Dead cells are food for bacteria. I didn't want to provide a free lunch for the bacteria that normally occupy our skin.

Second—and this did not make me popular with the OR staff—I did not allow street clothes into my OR.

What are you talking about? No one allows street clothes in the OR, right?

I disagree. Street clothes are allowed in the OR all the time. If someone wears their surgical scrubs around the hospital, then goes into the OR without changing into a clean pair, they have worn street clothes into the OR. If someone puts their scrubs on at home, drives to work, stops for coffee, walks around the hospital, then goes into the OR, they have worn street clothes into the OR.

I insisted that the entire staff change into fresh scrubs, caps, and shoe covers for every case. If I had three or four cases in a day, that meant changing scrubs et al between each case.

I was the only surgeon of any specialty at the USAF Hospital who insisted on that behavior. I am convinced that not wearing street clothes into the OR was a major contributor to my not having any wound infections.

I learned this tactic when I was a third-year medical student rotating on surgery. One week of my rotation was at the Shriners Burn Hospital. They not only required changing everything between cases, they also required showers between cases. Infection in the severely burned patients at the Shrine was devastating and sometimes fatal. The Shrine had very low infection rates.

Not wearing street clothes into the OR was, in my opinion, a major contributor to the Shrine's success. I believe *my* success was, probably in a major way, because of the policy I stole from the Shrine.

Crushed Upper Extremity

One day, while I was assigned to the USAF Hospital in the Azores, we got a message that a U.S. Navy sailor aboard a nuclear submarine had crushed his non-dominant left upper extremity in the sub's 3000-pound/square inch trash compactor. He was on his way to us and would reach us the next day.

Nuclear submarines were not allowed to surface in sight of land while on patrol. So, we arranged a time and place to meet the sub out of sight of the Azores.

This was an Air Force base, but we had some U.S. Army troops who oversaw the port and some Navy members who flew anti-submarine missions over the Atlantic Ocean in P3 Orion Anti-Submarine Warfare aircraft. The Air Force had the base, but no planes. The Army had some boats. And the Navy had planes. Go figure.

To get this sailor from the sub, two Army sergeants inflated a rubber Zodiac boat and attached two outboard motors. By setting the number of RPMs on the motors, using a stopwatch, and holding a steady compass heading, they could theoretically get to a predetermined point in the Atlantic beyond the horizon from land. There was no GPS.

So, I jumped into the Zodiac with the two Army sergeants, and off we went.

After quite a while we had reached our supposed meeting place. The sergeants stopped the motors. We bobbed up and down on the five-to-six-foot swells that we had been riding and fighting since we set off.

Soon, a large, black nuclear submarine surfaced directly beside us! Were we that good at finding our little plot of ocean? Doubtful. But submarine crews are pretty good at what they do.

The sailors aboard the sub manhandled their injured shipmate from the rolling, bobbing deck of the sub into our bobbing Zodiac. It would have been very easy to drop the man into the ocean. In other such transfers during my stay in the Azores, one sailor was dropped. One was crushed between the Zodiac and the sub. And one time the seas were so rough the injured man could not be off-loaded. One of our family physicians was in the Zodiac that day, and he climbed aboard the sub. The sub submerged and took our doctor away! Several days later we got a message he was ashore with the patient in Iceland!

But we got our man into the Zodiac and made a reciprocal course back to port. The sub silently submerged behind us.

When we got the man to the hospital, he was in a desperate condition. His left, non-dominant forearm was crushed and markedly swollen. He was in shock with falling blood pressure and rapid pulse and respirations. He had no pulses in his pale upper extremity. He had pain, was paralyzed, and had bizarre, electric-shock feelings called paresthesias in the extremity. Pain, Pale, Pulseless, Paresthetic, and Paralyzed. The five Ps of crush injuries.

The books said, given he had all five of the Ps and was more than seventy-two hours post injury, I should amputate.

But he was only nineteen years old and didn't want to lose his forearm and hand. And I didn't want to amputate.

So, we talked it over. I explained that the books said I should amputate, but if he was willing to take a chance, I would try to save his forearm and hand. I made sure he understood the odds were against success and that amputation was still going to be a possibility. We agreed to give saving the extremity a try.

Initially we had to get him tuned up to be well enough to go to the operating room. After a crush injury, there are *lots* of problems.

The crushed muscle releases proteins into the bloodstream that can clog the kidneys and cause them to fail. Chemicals from the crushed cells add potassium, calcium, and other electrolytes to the blood, creating marked abnormalities that can cause the heart to become irregular, or even stop. All those things had to be corrected. In this man's case, they had to be corrected very quickly as time was of the essence if there was even a remote chance of saving the limb. And saving the kidneys. And saving his life.

After our best effort to correct all his blood abnormalities, we took the man to the operating room, and the nurse anesthetist put him to sleep. The patient's heart did not skip a beat. So, it seemed we had gotten his blood chemistries under control.

I then did an anterior fasciotomy.

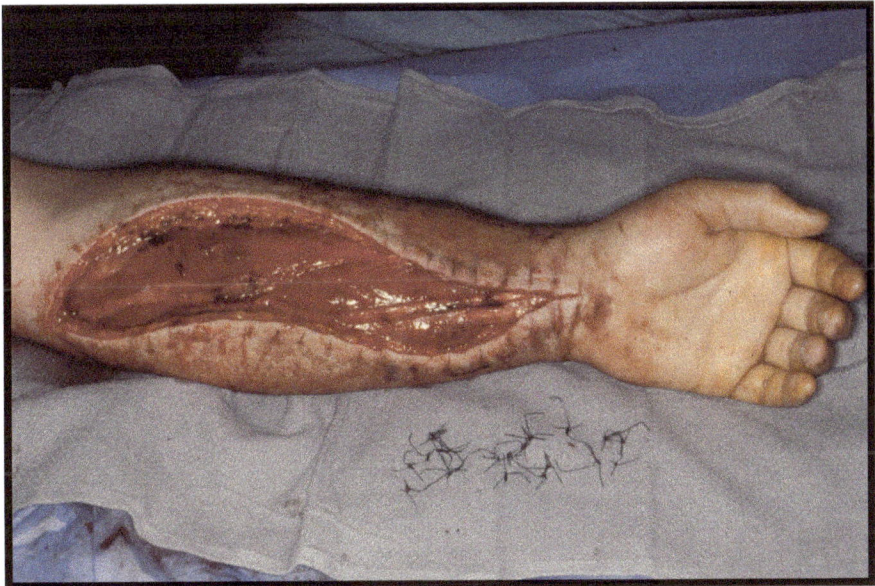

Anterior fasciotomy

The idea of fasciotomy is to cut the connective tissue that overlies the muscles that flex the wrist and fingers, allowing the swollen muscles to bulge through the cut and relieve pressure on the arteries. The hope is that by relieving the pressure, blood will again flow through the arteries. The fasciotomy did not work. No pulses.

So, then I did a posterior fasciotomy.

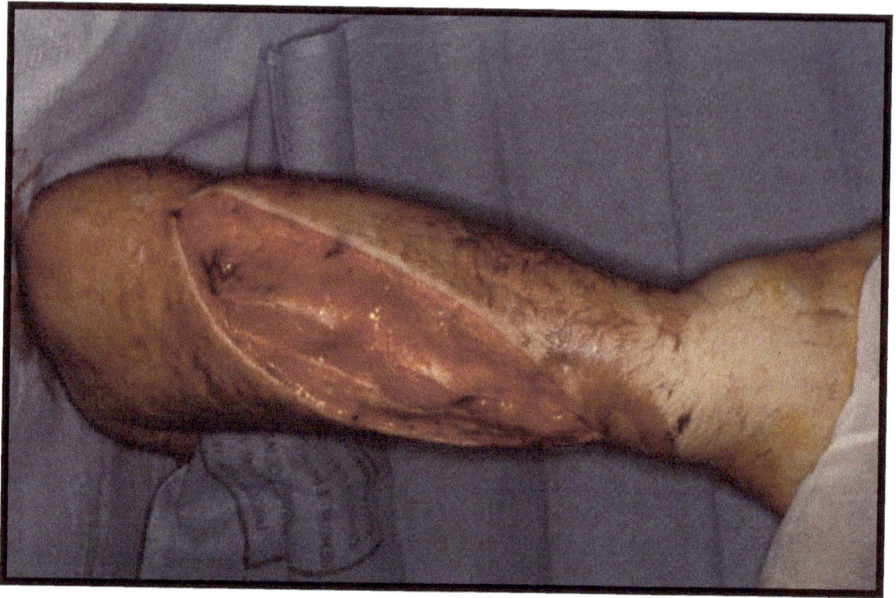

Posterior fasciotomy

Again, no return of pulses.

I did not take these pictures. They were taken at Andrews Air Force Base Hospital in Washington, D.C. days after the surgery we performed in the Azores. That is why there are stitches in the pictures.

So, I dissected down to the radial artery. There are three arteries that give blood supply to the hand: the radial, the ulnar, and the interosseous. All three arteries were clotted.

But, in nature's infinite wisdom, it takes only one patent artery to give complete blood supply to the hand, as all three arteries feed two arches in the hand from which all the other hand arteries arise.

I asked the nurse anesthetist to fully anticoagulate the patient. He responded he had never done that and did not know how. I was able to dredge up the formula from the depths of my memory, as I had not had to think about anticoagulating anyone since my residency. (Remember, this is before the internet.)

I then asked the circulating nurse to expose one of the patient's thighs and to surgically scrub, prep, and drape the thigh.

The assisting sergeant and I then moved from the forearm to the thigh, dissected down to the saphenous vein, and removed a segment of the vein. The saphenous vein is one of many veins draining the lower extremity and can safely be removed without any negative consequence to the leg or thigh.

We closed the thigh wound and took the vein segment back to the forearm. I removed the clotted segment of the radial artery and sewed the piece of saphenous vein in the artery's place. Of course, since veins in extremities have valves, it was important to make sure the vein had been placed such that the one-way valves allowed forward flow from the arm to the hand!

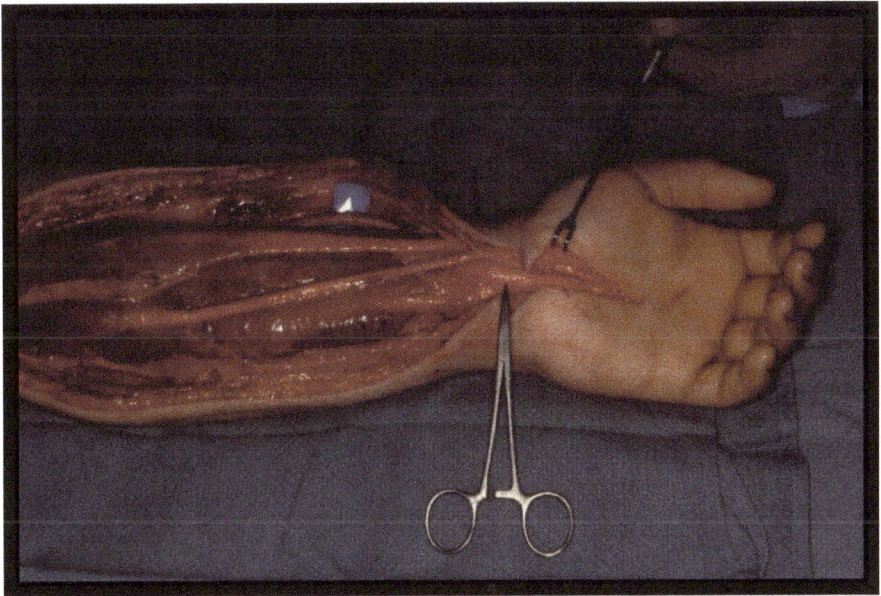

Saphenous vein graft

As soon as we took the clamps off the vessel, the hand pinked up.

The saphenous vein graft in place of the radial artery is under the blue tape in this picture. The clamp is pointing to the median nerve.

We closed the wounds with big, wide stitches.

The reason we did not do my normal cosmetic closure was that I planned to MedEvac this patient to Andrews Air Force Base Hospital as soon as we could so that the vascular surgeons could perform all additional surgeries he might need to try to save the forearm and hand. Big, wide stitches are what is called a "combat closure" and are intended to be removed as soon as the patient gets to the next higher level of care at a larger hospital.

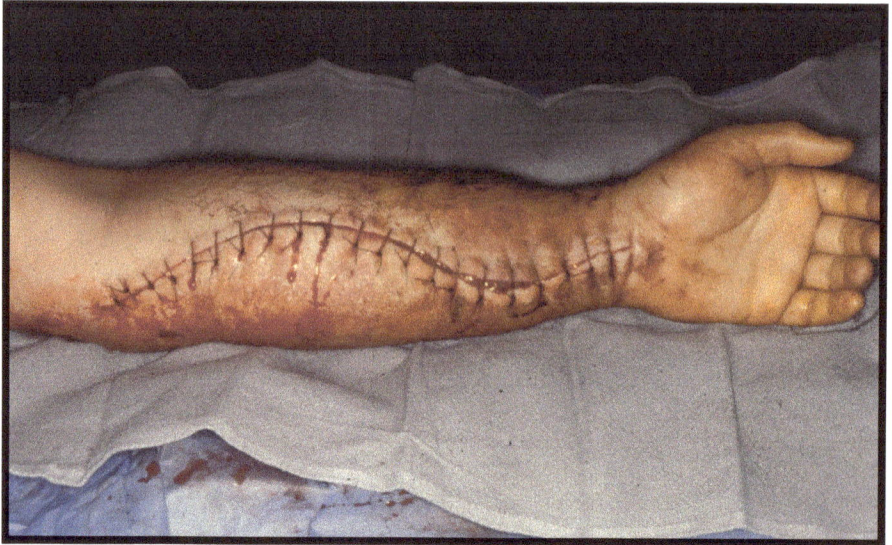

Combat closure

You can see that at Andrews, the surgeons exposed the patient's median nerve and found it to be intact.

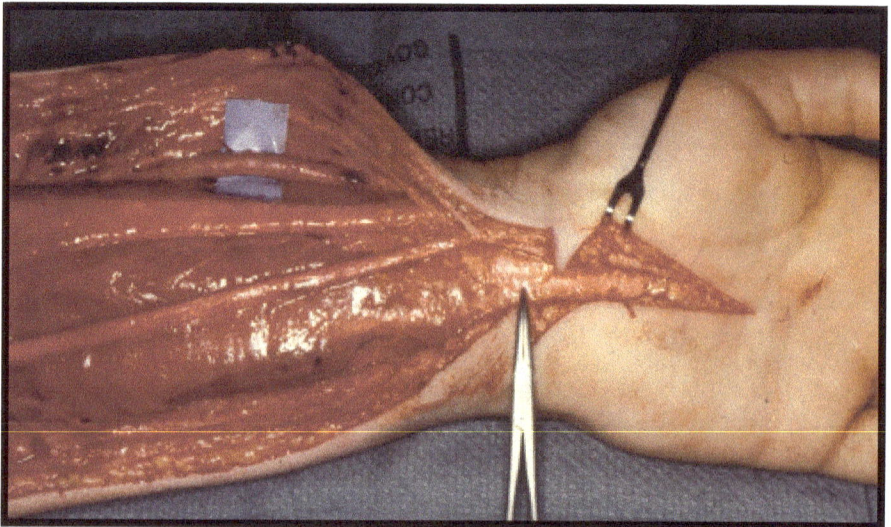

Median nerve exposure

The Andrews surgeons decided the vein graft we did was working and they did not do any further vascular work. However, by that time the patient was so swollen they could not close his wounds, so they had to skin graft him to get his wounds covered.

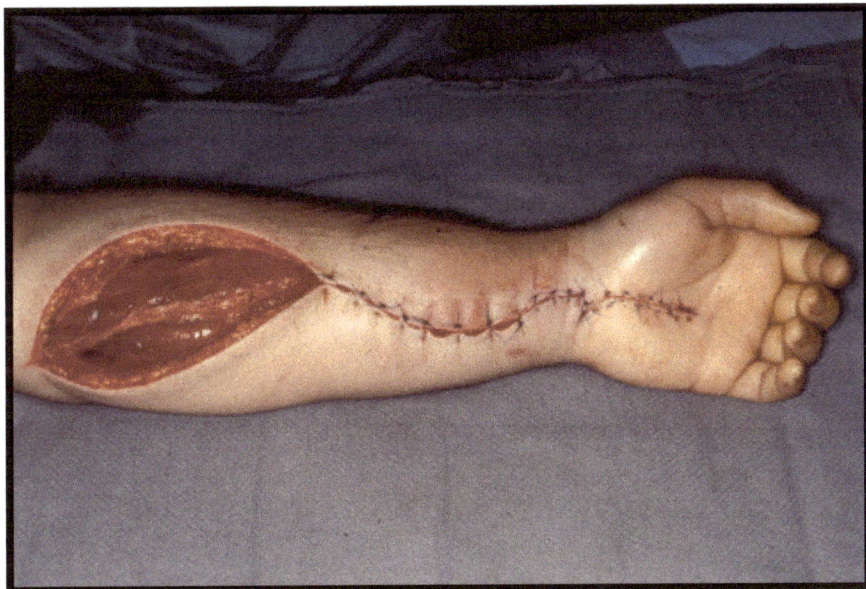

Anterior closure at Andrews—too swollen to completely close

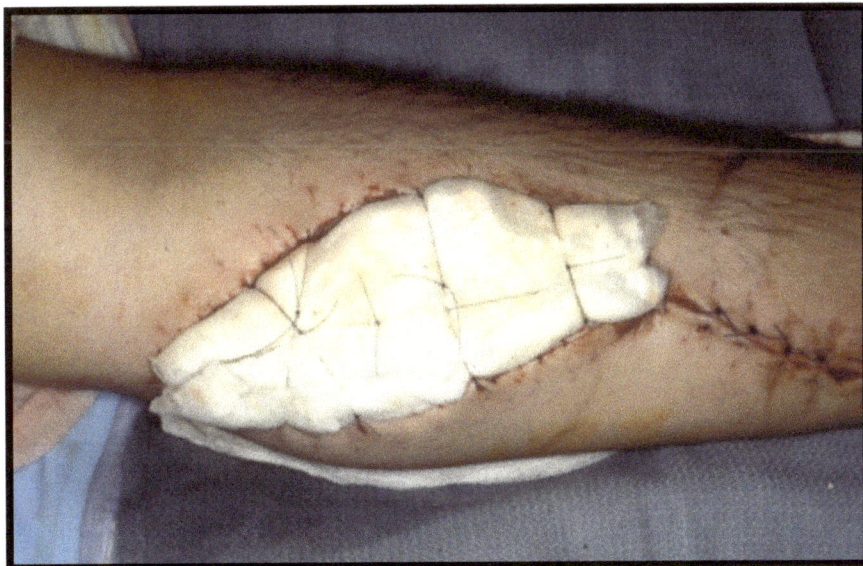

Bolster over anterior skin graft

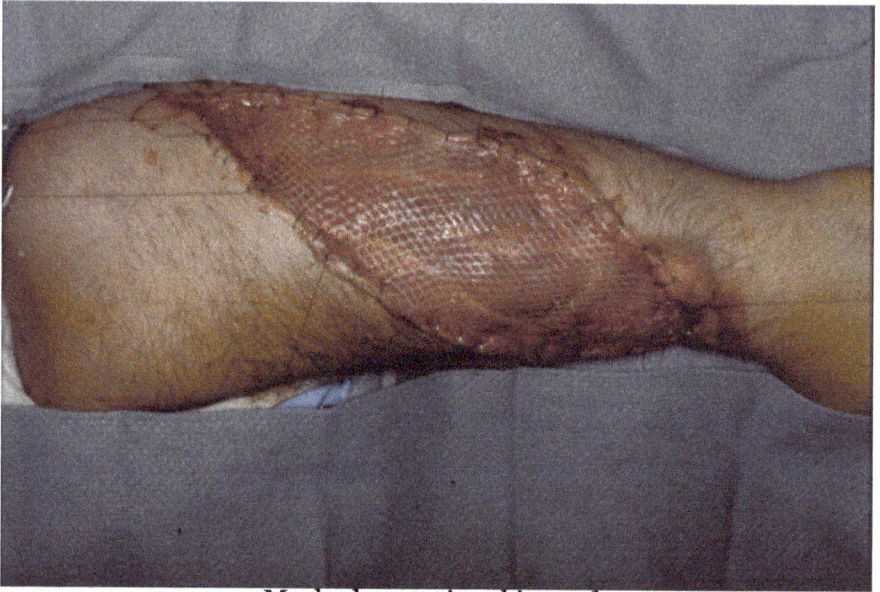
Meshed posterior skin graft

I heard that the patient subsequently recovered full use of his upper extremity. Was I correct not to amputate? Under most circumstances I was not correct. But this was a young, healthy person and there is no substitute for youth and health.

And, face facts, I was just lucky.

Breast Cancer

A very worried thirty-six-year-old woman came to my clinic at the USAF Academy Hospital for a breast mass. Her husband, a retired USAF sergeant, accompanied her. He had retired after twenty years of service because he enlisted when he was seventeen.

Indeed, upon examination, she had an easily palpable mass in her right breast. She had already had mammography, which had revealed diffuse microcalcifications throughout the breast and a normal appearing right breast.

I did a needle biopsy in the clinic which returned with malignant cells when pathology examined the specimen that afternoon.

Two days later, I again saw her in the clinic for a difficult conversation. This time, her husband did not accompany her.

She was young and pre-menopausal. Breast cancer is known to be diffusely found throughout the breast of a woman with a mass, and her breast was already showing mammogram evidence of diffuse disease. We discussed mastectomy (complete breast removal) as opposed to trying to just remove the mass and preserve the breast.

We also discussed the possibility of disease in her other breast. The literature at that time stated that the other breast had a ten percent chance of having cancer, and that the risk would go up one percent per year as long as she lived. That meant she would have a twenty percent or a one-in-five chance of cancer in the other breast when she was forty-six, and a thirty percent, or almost one-in-three chance of cancer in the other breast when she was fifty-six.

We talked about post-operative radiation and, if there was cancer found in her lymph nodes, chemotherapy.

After much discussion she agreed to come back in a few days with her decision. When she returned, she told me the only reasonable course, in her opinion, was to remove both breasts. I concurred.

After I did bilateral mastectomies, she had an uneventful postoperative course. Interestingly, her husband never was with her again for any of the visits except on the actual day of surgery. I never saw him visit her in the hospital when she was recovering. This was a definite red flag.

Her pathology revealed cancer diffusely through both breasts and she had positive lymph nodes in her right armpit.

I referred her to oncology who started her on chemotherapy. Additionally, I referred her to gynecology to discuss whether she should have her ovaries removed. Her cancer was estrogen-receptor positive, meaning cancer cells from the tumor grew aggressively in the lab when exposed to estrogen. Being pre-menopausal meant the patient was making estrogen from her ovaries which would encourage growth in any hidden metastases she might have.

Both gynecology and oncology advised her to have a complete hysterectomy. She had her ovaries and uterus removed.

About two months after her hysterectomy, the patient made an appointment to see me. She was not scheduled for any surgical follow-up, so I was surprised to see her on my schedule for the day. Her husband did not accompany her.

"How can I help you today?" I asked.

"Doctor Rizzo, what am I?"

"I'm sorry, I'm afraid I don't understand your question…"

"What am I?" she insisted, tears welling in her eyes.

"What do you mean?" I asked.

"Doctor, I have had my breasts removed. I have had my ovaries removed. I have had my uterus removed. I don't have my hair because of the chemo. I used to be a woman. What am I now?"

I must admit that was a question I had never heard before and had not anticipated. She clearly was much more troubled than I as a surgeon could address. We talked for a long time that morning, then I referred her to psychiatry so she could benefit from their expertise.

Then the presents started. She started leaving gifts for me, my wife, and my children with the clinic staff.

Soon after that her husband made an appointment to see me.

"How can I help you today?" I asked.

"I want to know if you're having an affair with my wife." He did not communicate that question/statement with any sort of politeness.

We also had a long talk about how much his wife was going through. I advised him that, no, I was not having an affair with his wife. I also advised him that she needed him more than ever before—both physically and psychologically.

Some weeks later, she left a message with the clinic staff that she and her husband were going to divorce.

I never saw or heard from her again.

She taught me a critically important lesson about the impact of what surgeons do. I had always prided myself on treating the whole patient and not just the disease. But accomplishing that goal requires a large team effort—and not just the surgeon and the OR team.

Infection above a Stone

One morning in the Azores, I was called to the ER by the family physician for a twenty-six-year-old wife of an active-duty Navy petty officer. She complained of two days of increasing left flank pain along with nausea, vomiting, fever, and chills. Her symptoms had increased to the point that she stated she was certain she was going to die.

Long before this, I had taken to heart a very real lesson: if a person tells you they are going to die you'd better listen. Because sometimes they die.

Since I was already in the hospital, I got to the ER in a couple of minutes to find the patient in acute distress, lying on the gurney, and obviously in severe pain.

She denied all other history or complaints. Her last menstrual period had been normal and ended one week prior to coming to the hospital.

Her blood pressure was 60/20, her pulse was 128, her respirations were 26 and panting, and her oral temperature was 104.6 degrees Fahrenheit. She was obviously in shock but had no obvious sign of trauma. Fortunately, her room air pulse oximeter was 98%, so she was oxygenating her blood—her lungs were probably working normally.

Upon physical exam, she had marked left costovertebral angle tenderness. That means when I tapped on the left side of her back at the angle between her lower ribs and spinal column, she was very tender. Costovertebral tenderness usually means there is something wrong with a kidney.

Her abdomen was soft but tender in the left upper quadrant.

The rest of her physical exam was normal.

Her labs revealed a white blood count of 20,800, which is double the upper limit of normal, along with an increase in neutrophils and lymphocytes. These values indicated she was infected somewhere. All the rest of her blood values were normal.

Her urine revealed too-numerous-to-count red blood cells and white blood cells, high levels of bacteria, and a specific gravity that implied dehydration.

Her abdominal X-rays revealed an approximately one-centimeter-diameter calcified mass on the left side of her abdomen at the level of the first lumbar vertebra.

I diagnosed a kidney stone with a urinary infection above the stone.

When this is seen it is almost always caused by *E.coli*, a bacterium from the colon that is a common cause of bladder infections in women. Her bladder infection had traveled through her bladder, up her ureters, and into her kidney. She was passing a kidney stone, the stone got stuck in the left ureter, and the infection was severely worsening above the stone.

This condition causes sepsis, which is why she was in shock. She was, in fact, dying.

There was no time to get a MedEvac plane to take her to a urologist in the United States. She would be dead long before we could get a plane to the Azores.

If we had had a urologist available, he or she would have passed a scope through her urethra, into her bladder, into and up her ureter, and visualized the stone. Through the scope, they would have passed a catheter up past the stone, inflated a balloon above the stone, and pulled the stone out by catching the stone with the balloon. We didn't have a urologist, a scope, or catheters.

So, after starting IVs to hydrate her and antibiotics to start killing the infection, I took her to the operating room.

I made a midline incision in her abdomen and dissected down just to the surface of the peritoneum, which is the lining of the abdominal cavity.

Normally, when making an incision to get into the abdomen, you cut right through the peritoneum. But the kidneys and ureters are behind the peritoneal cavity. So, I carefully dissected around the peritoneum, moving it to the right side of her body, exposing the area behind the peritoneum.

There was her ureter, and it looked red hot! It was obviously very swollen and inflamed. I cut her ureter open, and out popped a kidney stone, followed by a huge amount of pus and urine.

The nurse anesthetist exclaimed that her pulse, which had been racing even under general anesthesia, immediately came down to normal after the pus was drained.

Now I had a problem.

If you sew a ureter together it will scar closed. Then urine would be unable to drain from the kidney into the bladder, and the kidney would die. The only way to close a ureter is over a stint or a catheter. But I didn't have any of those.

So, I completely transected the ureter and brought both ends out through a second incision I made in the abdomen. I sewed both ends to the skin and secured them as ureterostomies.

After irrigating the area to clean up the pus and urine, I closed the patient and put a colostomy bag over the ureterostomies I had created.

In the recovery room, the patient's temperature returned to normal—draining the pus and backed-up urine, along with the antibiotics, were doing the job of defeating the sepsis that was trying to kill her.

We called for a MedEvac plane, and, within forty-eight hours she was at Andrews Air Force Base Hospital in Washington, D.C.

About two weeks later, I was on the ward seeing a patient I had operated on when the patient came walking down the hall.

"You're back!" I exclaimed.

"Yes, I'm all better!"

"What did they do for you at Andrews?"

"They took me to the OR and closed my ureters over a stint. Two days ago, they pulled the stint out and here I am!"

"I'm so glad to see you! Thank you for coming in!"

Amazingly, I didn't see her again for the rest of her husband's assignment in the Azores. I never heard from the urologists at Andrews, so I guess doing a ureterostomy as if it were a colostomy worked out.

Saphenous Vein Thrombosis

One Friday afternoon at the USAF Academy Hospital in Colorado Springs, Colorado, a thirty-nine-year-old family practice physician assistant decided to drive from Colorado Springs to Atlanta, Georgia. He started his trip after his clinic was done, around 5:00 pm. He had to be back in Colorado Springs for duty in his clinic at 8:00 am on Monday morning.

He must drive about 1,400 miles each way—2,800 miles, have time to do whatever he wanted to do, and get back to duty in sixty-three hours. He had to be in the car for about twenty-one driving hours each way, or forty-two hours. That left twenty-one hours to get three night's sleep and do whatever he wanted to do in Atlanta.

To jump ahead: he became my patient, and he never told me why he made this trip. I suspect it had to do with a female.

When the PA got back, he did not report to his clinic on Monday morning. Instead, he came to my surgery clinic with a painful, swollen left lower extremity. Upon examination, he had an easily palpable (able to be felt) clot in his saphenous vein. Forty-two hours of driving, with few or no stops to rest or walk around, had caused this long vein to clot on his left side.

The clot was palpable from this medial malleolus (middle ankle bone) to just above his left knee.

The saphenous vein is a superficial vein. Normally, doctors worry about a deep vein clotting, then a piece of clot breaking off and traveling through the heart and into the lungs. This is a pulmonary embolus and has the potential to be fatal. The risk was still there from the superficial saphenous, but the risk was less than from a deep vein.

I asked the PA what he wanted to do. "I don't want surgery, and I don't want to be admitted," he said. Which made me wonder why he came to me in the surgery clinic.

"OK," I said. "You understand there is a risk of some of this clot breaking loose and going to your lungs."

"Yup," he said.

So, we agreed to put him on an anticoagulant, placed him on bed rest with his lower extremity elevated, and I set him up for a visit the next day.

The next morning, he appeared in my clinic. The clot was now palpable to mid-thigh. I told him I was more worried than the day before about a pulmonary embolus. "I don't want surgery, and I don't want to be admitted," he said.

Making sure he understood the risk, I agreed to give him one more day of anticoagulant, rest, and elevation. But I didn't like it.

The next day, Wednesday, the PA appeared in my clinic. The clot was now palpable in the upper third of his thigh.

The saphenous vein dives into the deep venous system in the groin. The risk of a pulmonary embolus was now undeniable.

In the military, a medical order is a military order. So, I didn't give the PA a choice. I told him we were going to the operating room to prevent a pulmonary embolus and save his life.

I called the OR and spoke with the charge nurse. "Major," I said, "I need to bring over an emergency case."

"No problem," she said. "I have one open room and the other seven are going. What is the emergency?"

"It's a vein case."

She said, in her best, sternest, Air Force major charge nurse voice, "There's no such thing as a vein emergency."

"I didn't think so, either, but there is now."

She had the circulating nurse pull the instruments from my vein stripping card. Every surgeon had a card for each of the kinds of cases they performed. That card had the surgeon's preferred instruments. A vein stripping is a barbaric operation that, thankfully, is not done anymore. It involved ripping the saphenous vein from its place using a hook and a long plastic tube. But, of course, the card also had basic instruments such as a knife, forceps, and hemostats.

We got to the OR and prepped the PA's entire left lower extremity. I incised from groin to ankle, exposing the clotted, varicose saphenous vein in its entirety. I already knew he had varicose veins and that his clotted saphenous was varicose. A varicose vein is a twisted, swollen vein that has multiple failed valves.

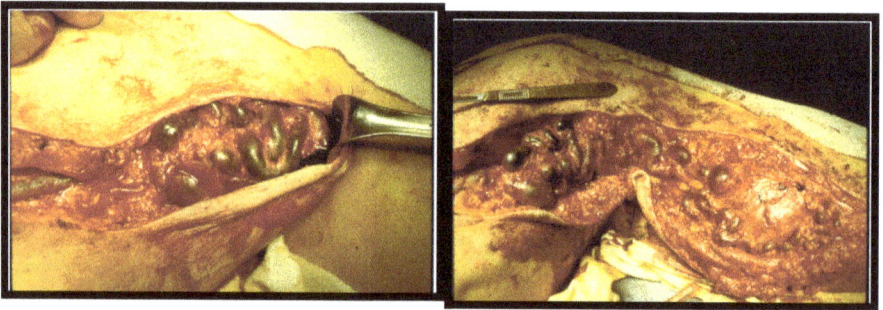

Clotted, very tortuous varicose vein

All his twisted varicosities were clotted. You can see how large the vein is in the thigh as compared with my finger:

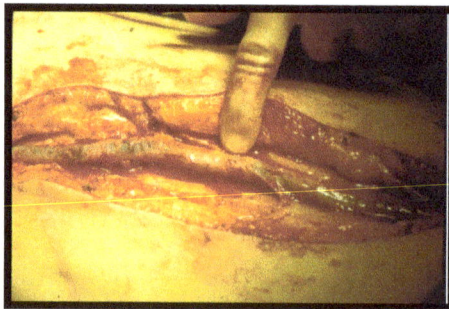

Clotted saphenous vein compared to my finger

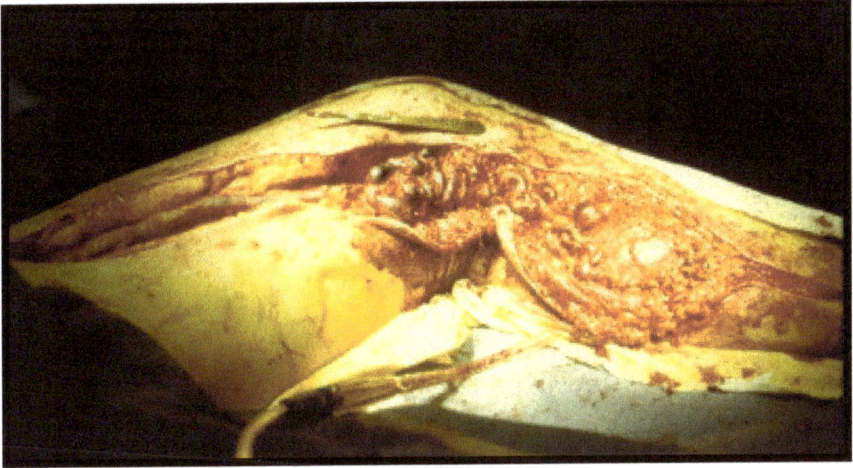

Entire vein exposed

We removed the entire saphenous vein.

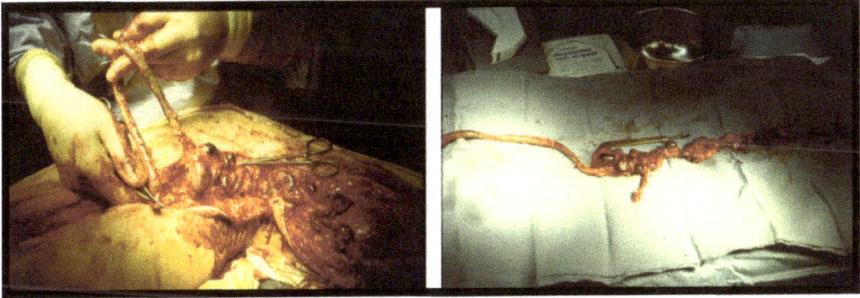

Removing the vein and vein stretched out on back table

I closed him up, and he had an uneventful recovery.

People do just fine without their saphenous veins, as the lower extremities have both a deep and superficial system of veins. A portion of the saphenous is what I removed to replace the crushed radial artery in the sailor from the submarine described elsewhere in this book. Saphenous veins are used for coronary artery bypass surgery.

What was amazing was how busy my OR became during the case. Literally every surgeon in the hospital somehow had a reason to come into my OR, take a look and ask, "Rizzo, just what the hell are you doing?" In my general surgery room, I was visited by orthopedics, urology, gynecology, the other general surgeons, and even a dermatologist (who had no business in the OR at all)!

To reiterate, the PA never told me why he made the trip to Atlanta. I hope it was worth it.

Right Upper Quadrant Pain

One day, in my surgery clinic at the U.S. Air Force Hospital, I saw the forty-two-year-old wife of an active-duty Air Force sergeant who complained of several months of right upper quadrant abdominal pain radiating straight through to her back. She said it was constant but much worse when she ate fried or fatty foods.

This is the classic story of gallbladder disease. In fact, this patient had all the Fs of gallbladder disease: "female, forties, fat, and fertile."

She was clearly female. She was in her forties. She weighed 230 pounds and was five-foot-six-inches tall. She had had four pregnancies and deliveries.

She had no previous surgeries. Her meds included birth control pills, an antihypertensive for high blood pressure, and a statin drug for high cholesterol.

Her family physician had ordered a gallbladder ultrasound that was interpreted by the radiologist as "normal."

She had a perfect story for gallbladder disease, and her physical exam revealed tenderness in the abdominal right upper quadrant consistent with gallbladder disease.

But she had a normal gallbladder ultrasound.

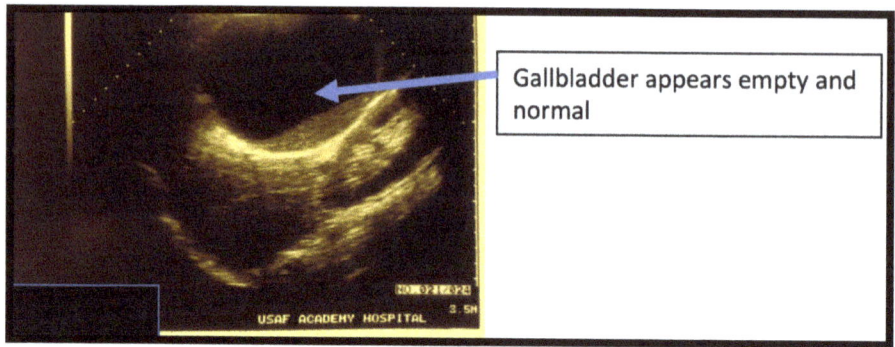

Gallbladder appears normal on ultrasound

At the time I saw this patient, the test that is now considered the gold standard for gallbladder disease had not yet been invented. That test is a HIDA scan. HIDA stands for Hepatobiliary Iminodiacetic Acid scan. In this test, the patient is given a radioactive dye that collects in the gallbladder. Then the patient is given an injection of cholecystokinin (CCK). CCK is a hormone produced by the small intestines that causes the gallbladder to contract. The patient is placed under the gamma camera that can see the radioactive dye in the gallbladder, the CCK is administered, and the amount of dye that is ejected from the gallbladder is observed. If the ejection is greater than thirty to thirty-five percent, the gallbladder is considered normal.

But, as I said, the HIDA scan had not yet been invented. All we had to go on was her history and physical findings along with the ultrasound.

Because the ultrasound was negative, I had to consider what else could be causing her pain. On the list of differential diagnoses were pancreatitis, peptic ulcer, diverticulitis, or some other intra-abdominal pathology that would be rare or unusual.

I repeated her ultrasound, and it was again negative per radiology. It looked exactly like the first ultrasound.

Her pancreas lab tests were normal. X-rays of her abdomen were normal. Her pregnancy test was negative. Everything I could think of to check was normal.

And the patient was in considerable pain all the time, but especially after eating. By this time her pain increased after eating anything at all.

The problem at that time was that taking someone to the operating room to remove a gallbladder was a big deal. Laparoscopic surgery had not yet been invented. Removing a gallbladder required a big abdominal incision. Operating on an overweight person was difficult and had an increased risk of postoperative complications. She was probably looking at a two-week stay in the hospital, even if she did not have any complications.

Further, the standard of surgical care was only to operate if someone had a positive ultrasound.

One of my fellow surgeons at the USAF Academy told me if I took her to the OR and removed a normal gallbladder, it would be considered malpractice.

She and I talked it over. I told her she was the textbook picture of gallbladder disease even though her ultrasound was negative. She insisted she could not live with the pain she was having. So, I bit the bullet and scheduled her for surgery.

As soon as she was put to sleep in the OR, and before I made the skin incision, the chief surgeon came into the room and said, "Rizzo, this better be a sick gallbladder or you're going to get sued." He reminded me that, while active-duty members could not sue individual physicians for malpractice (they must sue the Air Force), dependents certainly can. He went on to say that if asked, he would encourage such a suit because "It is wrong to take out a gallbladder if the ultrasound is negative."

With those words of encouragement from my colleague and superior officer, I made the skin incision and wrestled through the layers of fat to get her gallbladder out.

Once the gallbladder was out, I put it on the back table and cut it open. It was tightly packed with stones.

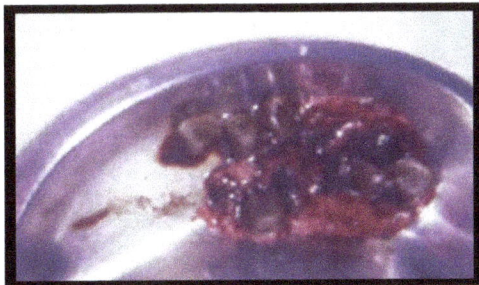

Gallbladder opened—packed with stones

The reason the ultrasound was negative was that the gallbladder was so tightly packed with stones, there was no space between any of them to cause a shadow.

She had an uneventful post-op recovery—thank goodness.

Now that the HIDA scan is a thing, we know that people can have sick gallbladders without any stones at all. If the ejection fraction on the HIDA is less than thirty percent, the gallbladder is sick and needs to come out.

Sick gallbladders can cause the patient to become septic. Sepsis is the leading cause of death in ICUs in the United States. So, getting a sick gallbladder out is important.

But, at the time I saw this woman, the criteria were stones or no stones.

Abdominal Pain

I was called to the USAF Hospital ER for a fifty-eight-year-old wife of a retired USAF officer complaining of six hours of acute onset mid-epigastric pain.

Acute onset abdominal pain can have many causes. In the midepigastric region, one had to think about the liver, gallbladder, pancreas, stomach, small intestine, large intestine, and other organs that don't normally live in the midepigastric region but could have wandered there.

This woman stated she had no appetite—making me immediately think of appendicitis. Except the appendix is nowhere near the midepigastric region, and she had previously had her appendix out.

Next, the gallbladder came to mind, but she had had that out, also.

She was fifty-eight, so pregnancy was unlikely. She had had three pregnancies and three deliveries in the past and was postmenopausal.

Her only other medical history was high blood pressure, for which she was under good control on medication. Her vital signs included a slightly high blood pressure, pulse, and respirations, but those were likely due to her level of pain—which was high.

Sometimes women with heart attacks can present as mid-epigastric pain instead of chest pain. But her ECG was normal, as was her chest X-ray.

Her labs revealed a white blood count of 11,400 with increased neutrophils. Those findings clearly said she had inflamation or an infection going on.

Her abdominal X-ray revealed a fixed loop of small intestine in the midepigastrium. So, it appeared her small intestine had stopped working and bacteria there were producing gas that was visible on X-ray.

Her entire physical exam was normal except for her abdomen. She was markedly tender when I pressed on her abdomen, and she was guarding. Guarding is when the abdominal muscles go into spasm to keep the abdomen from moving. It's the body's way of trying to protect itself from pain. The organs in the abdominal cavity are innervated by spinal nerves that have branches to the overlying muscles and skin. When there is an intra-abdominal crisis that stimulates the spinal nerves, the branches to the overlying muscles stimulate the muscles into spasm.

When one sees an elevated white count with a left shift (increased neutrophils) along with guarding, it's considered an emergency. So, I took her to the OR to explore her abdomen.

She had three diverticula of her small intestine, and all three were inflamed.

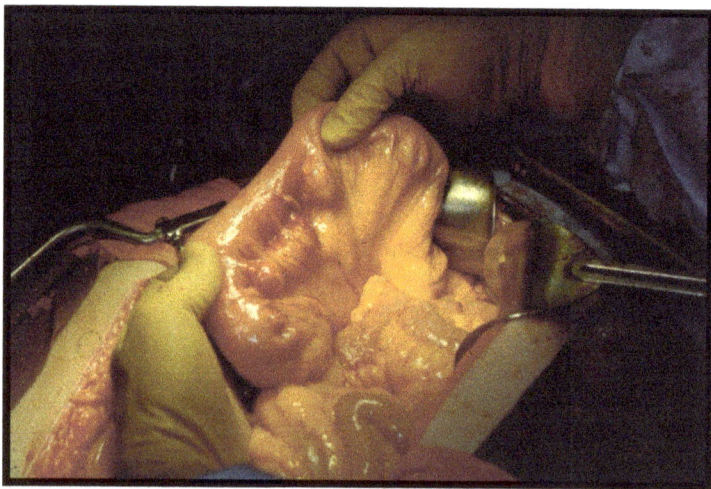

Three inflamed small intestinal diverticula

Diverticula are hernias of the intestinal wall. They are common in the large intestine. I had never heard of, or read about, diverticula of the small intestine.

When you're in the OR with someone's life in your hands, it's a good idea to have previously seen, read about, and studied what you find. One of the reasons surgery residency takes five years is that you have a chance to see a wide range of pathology. It's a bad, bad feeling to find something in the OR you have never seen or heard of before.

So, I had the circulating nurse call the other three staff surgeons and asked them to come to the OR.

When they arrived, they looked and said, "Wow! Small intestine diverticula. I've never seen that before!"

They were not going to be any help.

"What are you going to do, Rizzo?"

I considered removing the entire segment of small intestine and hooking the two ends back together. It was straightforward and usually had a good outcome. But the intestine from which these diverticula were suspended looked grossly completely normal. I hated to take out normal intestine if it was unnecessary.

I said, "I think I'm going to take out the diverticula and close her up. If she doesn't do well, I guess I can go back in and resect that segment of small intestine."

"Are you sure? You may be dooming her to a second operation when you could just resect now and be done with it."

"I know but look at her small intestine. It looks perfectly normal. I hate to take out normal organs. I'm going to take a chance."

"OK, Rizzo, it's your funeral."

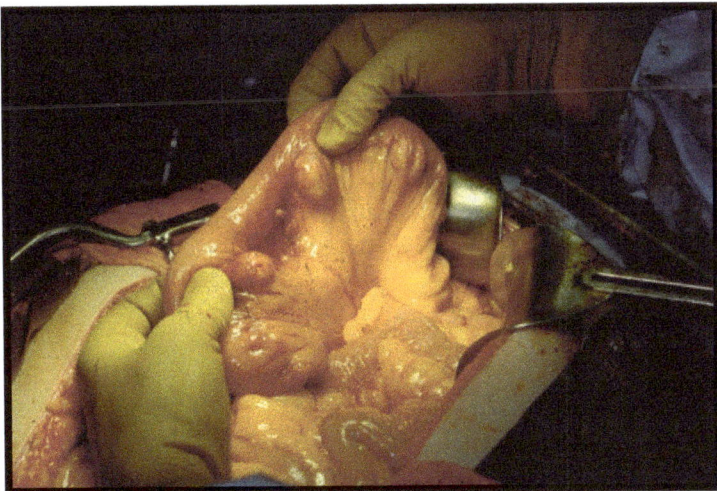

The center diverticulum has been removed

I tied off the stump, then repeated the process on the other two tics.

Post-operatively, the woman had an uneventful course. Her white blood count came back to normal, her vital signs normalized, she got her appetite back, and she was discharged in a few days.

Did I do the right thing? That's the problem with a case like this. If you go by outcome, then the answer is yes, I did the right thing. But you always wonder, "Was I just lucky?"

Sat on a Knife

In the Azores, the Navy had P3 Orion antisubmarine warfare planes. They flew antisub missions over the Atlantic pretty much around the clock. That meant there were numerous sailors assigned to the Azores whose mission was support and maintenance of the P3s.

One afternoon, one of our three family practice docs called me to the ER for a stab wound to the chest.

My family's quarters were only a couple of blocks from the hospital. However, the Azores is an archipelago of volcanic islands. Those couple of blocks were up a hill that was inclined about forty-five degrees at its shallowest and about sixty degrees at its steepest. So, it took me a few minutes to get there.

When I arrived, I found a female Navy petty officer with a stab wound through her utility uniform and into her chest. It appeared she had been stabbed in the back while at work.

I asked her what had happened. "I sat on a knife," she said.

This is the classic response of someone who doesn't want to tell you the truth. I assumed she was protecting someone, or she was so afraid of whoever stabbed her she was protecting herself by not telling me what really happened.

I did my best to explore the wound in the ER. We got a chest X-ray, which of course we had to read ourselves, and it did not appear she had a pneumothorax (collapsed lung). I anesthetized the wound with injections of a local anesthetic and tried to explore it to see if it went all the way to the pleura (covering of the lung). If the wound was that deep, she might develop a pneumothorax over the next minutes or hours. But the wound was too deep to get a good look.

I called the nurse anesthetist and the family practice doc, and I took her to the operating room. There I opened the wound and found it went down to a rib, taking a chunk out of the rib, but miraculously avoided going deeper. No collapsed lung in her future.

After cleaning the wound, I closed her up.

Later, after she recovered, I again asked her what had happened. "I sat on a knife," she said.

She obviously did not want to tell me what happened. But this time I was persistent. Once she realized I was not trying to get her into any trouble with her Navy command, she told me she always carried her lunch to work in a backpack. The lunch that day was a bread roll, some meat and cheese, and a foot-long knife to cut the food. She said she had the backpack on and flopped down on a park bench that was in the P3 hangar. When she hit the back of the bench, the knife penetrated the backpack and her back.

OK, I thought, *that's a pretty good story.* But I was still suspicious she was either protecting someone who had stabbed her or was afraid of being stabbed again.

I examined her backpack. Sure enough, it contained the food she described and had a hole in it consistent with a knife penetration.

I went down to the hangar and found the bench. Her injury could have happened just the way she described. One of her shipmates, who was there, told me she saw the accident and that my patient sat on a knife and stabbed herself in the back.

So, the patient was telling the truth, although her story was exactly what someone would have said in much more suspicious circumstances.

Moral of the story? I was still a surgeon who had done a residency in a major metropolitan city and to whom thousands of lies had been told to cover up something or someone. But I was now a surgeon who couldn't simply assume everyone was lying to him all the time.

Face Trauma

An eighteen-year-old active-duty airman was deployed to the Azores during Desert Storm directly after completing basic training. A sizable air refueling wing had been deployed to the Azores and this airman was part of that wing.

In the lead-up to Desert Storm, numerous fighter aircraft had to get from the U.S. to the Middle East. These aircraft did not have the range to cross the Atlantic. So, they would launch heading east from the U.S. east coast while refuelers from the wing in the Azores launched heading west. The refuelers would then air refuel the fighters and "drag them" across the Atlantic Ocean, refueling the fighters as needed until the flight reached Europe. The fighters would then meet refuelers based in Europe who dragged them to the Middle East, while the Azores refuelers headed back to the Azores for maintenance, rest, and refueling.

The airman in question was the youngest and lowest-ranking person in the refueling wing.

A bunch of his older enlisted brethren decided one night to "make this airman a man" by getting him drunk for the first time in his life.

Not the best idea.

When the airman staggered to the latrine to vomit, he pushed his face through a glass shelf that was over the sink. His highly intoxicated colleagues brought him to the ER and the family physician on duty called me.

He was in good health with no known medical problems and took no meds. He was able to be roused to answer questions, but it was clear he had no idea where he was or what was happening to him. He was extremely intoxicated.

Other than the extensive lacerations of his face, his physical exam was unremarkable, as were his labs. It did not appear his eyeballs had been involved in the lacerations.

However, I was unable to determine if he had fractured any facial bones or if he may have had a sinus punctured by the glass-shelf shards. This was the Azores, so a CT scan was unavailable. All we had was our physical findings and plain X-rays which we had to read ourselves.

The fingers in the following lateral facial view are mine. The airman was so drunk he could not follow instructions to hold his head still, so I had to hold him in place.

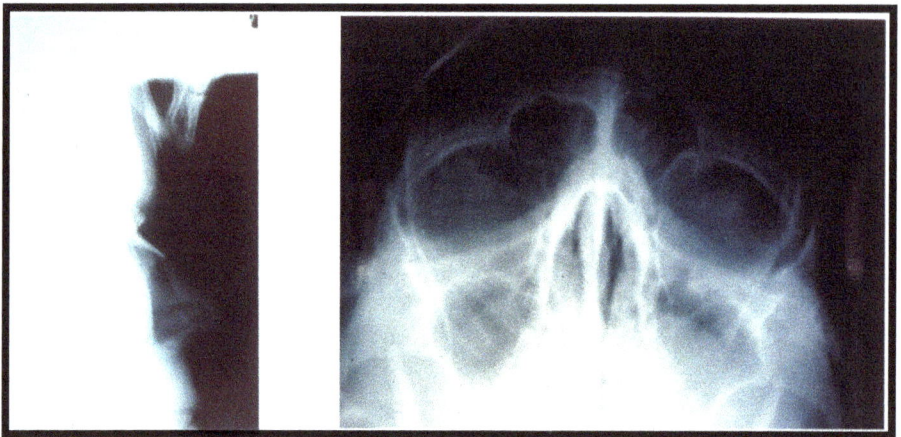

Facial X-rays demonstrating nasal fracture and no blood in maxillary sinus

The Water's view did not demonstrate blood in his frontal or maxillary sinuses, so I decided his only fracture was to his nasal septum.

Because the wound was so extensive, I decided to take him to the OR to explore and repair it. I simply could not see trying to use local anesthetic in the ER for wounds that severe.

Of course, given his inebriated state, the patient was not NPO (nothing by mouth), so our nurse anesthetist had to take special care to keep him from aspirating.

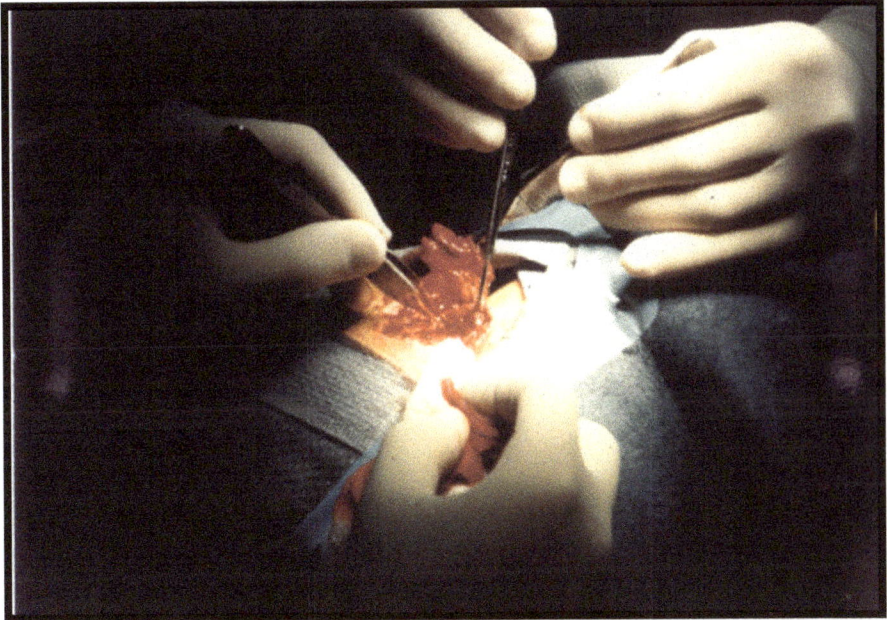

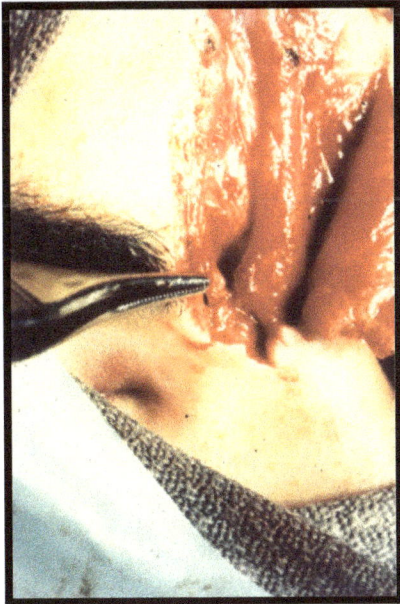

Facial exploration and lacerated lacrimal duct

(The hemostat in the photo is pointing to a lacrimal duct that was cut and needed to be repaired.)

Every time a person blinks, tears are washed from the upper, outer corner of his or her eye, across the front of the eye, and are drained via the lacrimal ducts into the nose. When one cries, he or she gets a runny nose because one makes excess tears that drain into your nose. That runny nose is tears. Eventually, if a person cries enough, the lacrimal ducts cannot handle the volume of tears, and some leak out and down one's face.

Failure to recognize the ductal injury and repair it could have left this patient with a lifetime of tears running down his cheek every time he blinked.

This airman had been in the Azores three days when the event happened. His post-op course included being MedEvac'd to the States. His war was over.

Although I tried to find out, I never discovered if there was punishment for the sergeants who got this airman drunk, causing a lifetime of scarring.

Nipple Bleeding

One day in the Azores, a twenty-three-year-old woman came to my clinic accompanied by her active-duty USAF airman husband and her three-month-old baby.

The patient and her husband were clearly anxious.

"How can I help you today?"

"I'm pretty sure I'm giving cancer to my baby!" The woman began to cry. Her husband was trying to hold it together but was also visibly upset.

"How are you giving cancer to your baby?"

"I'm breastfeeding and now there's blood in the milk! Blood in the milk has to be from breast cancer! I'm killing my baby!"

I did my best to reduce the extreme tension in the room and asked if I could examine the patient's breast.

Her breast was engorged with milk. "Are you able to show me the blood?" I asked.

The patient went directly to one of her left breast's milk glands, pressed on it, and, while she expressed milk, there was also a small amount of blood from one of the milk ducts.

Women all have about the same number of milk glands—usually between twenty-five and thirty in each breast. The number of milk glands and their size is remarkably consistent from one woman to another. The reason women have different-sized breasts is due to the amount of fat that surrounds the milk glands. Of course, when a woman is breastfeeding, her milk glands enlarge and become engorged with milk.

I told the woman that breast cancer was unlikely in her case. "Only about ten percent of breast cancers present as a mass that produces blood from the nipple," I said. Also, you are only twenty-three. So, you are nowhere near the age group in which we would expect breast cancer."

The woman and her husband were only minimally reassured.

"This is most likely a benign adenoma. An adenoma is a benign (I kept repeating the word benign) tumor of a gland. Benign adenomas can bleed."

"Are you sure it's not cancer?"

"The only way to be completely sure is to take the mass out. We can do that in such a way that you will be able to continue to breastfeed," I said.

"I want it out right now!"

I called the OR, and we scheduled her for the first day her husband would be able to accompany her and take care of the baby.

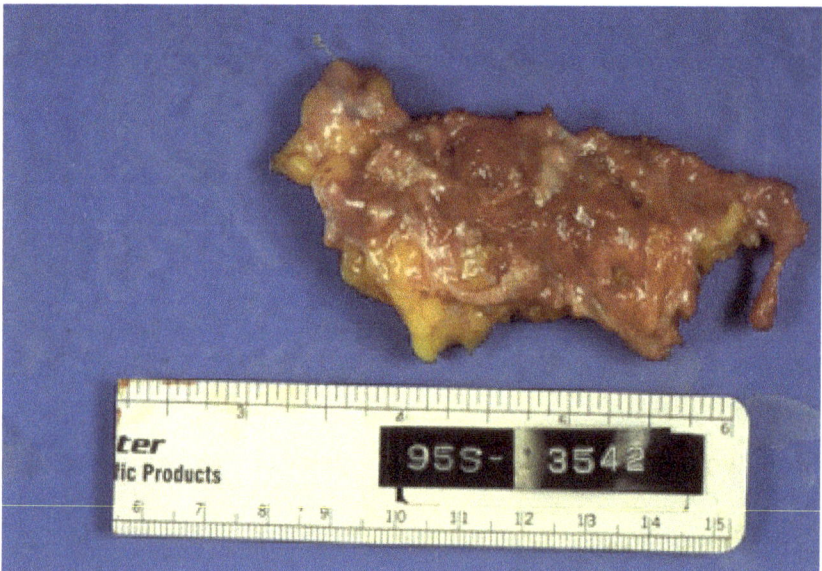

Fat-covered mammary gland and duct

I made a circumareolar incision, meaning an incision around the areola, the pigmented part of the breast that surrounds the nipple. I was then able to dissect down to the milk gland in question, which was easy to find because when I pressed on it, blood came out of her nipple. I removed only that gland and its duct with some surrounding breast fat.

I closed her up, and she was able to breastfeed in the recovery room.

Pathology came back with "benign adenoma."

After removing her sutures, I never saw her, her husband, or the baby again. That is how successful surgeries go: you can make patients better and they get on with their lives.

Wrist Laceration

The family physician covering the ER in the Azores called me to see an active-duty Navy petty officer with a wrist laceration. He described the laceration as a "little thing," but said he was having trouble evaluating the patient and wondered if I would take a look to see if any deep structures had been involved.

When I got to the ER, I found a twenty-eight-year-old who was exceptionally intoxicated. He was so drunk he could not speak. He was, in fact, unconscious and barely responsive. He could not answer questions or cooperate in any way with his exam.

I could see why the family doc had been unable to evaluate him.

Several drunken shipmates brought him in and slurred that he had been trying to wash a glass and cut his wrist.

This story did not seem true.

The patient was married, but his wife was at home, had not come to the ER with the patient, and was refusing to help or answer questions.

Because the patient could not answer questions, his past medical history was completely unknown.

His vital signs were stable. He was unable to move his hand or fingers, unable to make a fist, unresponsive to pinprick when sticking his fingers— but it was impossible to determine if that was because he had cut tendons and nerves in his wrist or simply because of his alcohol anesthesia. He had strong pulses in his wrist and his capillary refill was normal (when I pressed on the nails, the nailbed got pale; when I released the pressure on the nail the nailbed pinked up immediately). So, we knew he had a good blood supply to his hand.

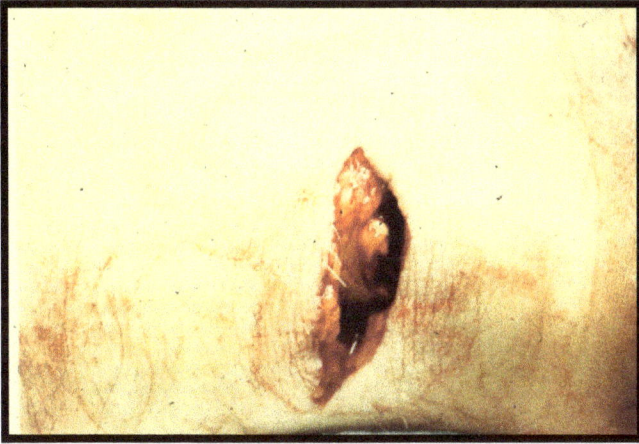

Wrist laceration as it appeared in the Emergency Room

Our concerns were whether he had cut his tendons to his hand and fingers, cut the nerves controlling his hand muscles and providing sensation to his hand, possibly cut an artery that was clamped down but would bleed later, and whether this had been a suicide attempt.

I called in our nurse anesthetist. Clearly this patient was not NPO, which is a real concern when taking someone to the OR for general anesthesia. As mentioned earlier in this book, NPO stands for *nolo per oris*, which is Latin for nothing by mouth. We want people to be NPO before general anesthesia because when you wake up someone from anesthesia and remove their breathing tube, they tend to gag and vomit. If the patient's stomach is empty, they have nothing to vomit. We don't want them to vomit because vomiting when recovering from anesthesia can lead to aspiration. Aspiration is when something other than air goes down the trachea into the lungs. Stomach contents are acidic. Aspirating stomach contents leads to aspiration pneumonia which has a fifteen percent mortality rate.

Surgeons want patients to be NPO.

The reason for considering taking this patient to the OR with the risk of aspiration was that if he cut the tendons in his wrist, they can retract high up into the proximal forearm making it difficult to repair the tendons. The other reason was that there are three major arteries in the wrist. We knew he had a good radial pulse, but did not know about the other two. If one of those arteries had been cut, it was not bleeding now—arteries tend to go into spasm when cut—but the spasm would eventually relax, and he could bleed several hours later.

Basically, I felt we should explore the patient's forearm and take the risk of aspiration. The nurse anesthetist concurred and would take appropriate precautions to preclude aspiration from happening.

Of course, this patient could not give us surgical consent, being unconscious from alcohol. His wife continued to be uncooperative.

I wrote on the chart that this was an emergency, and I was taking the patient to the OR using the concept of implied consent. Implied consent is a best guess that a patient, in an emergency situation, would consent to surgery if he or she had been able to.

***

In the OR, I opened the forearm to discover the patient had cut every one of the tendons that flexed his fingers.

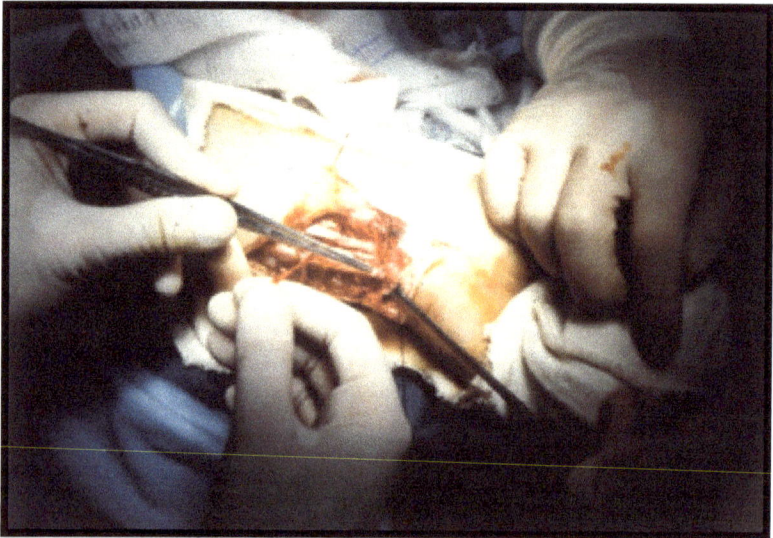

Repairing the flexor tendons in the forearm

It took us four hours to repair all his tendons. Fortunately, there was no sign of arterial or nerve damage.

I had opened the patient's forearm by extending the edges of his laceration, creating triangular flaps resulting in an angular closure.

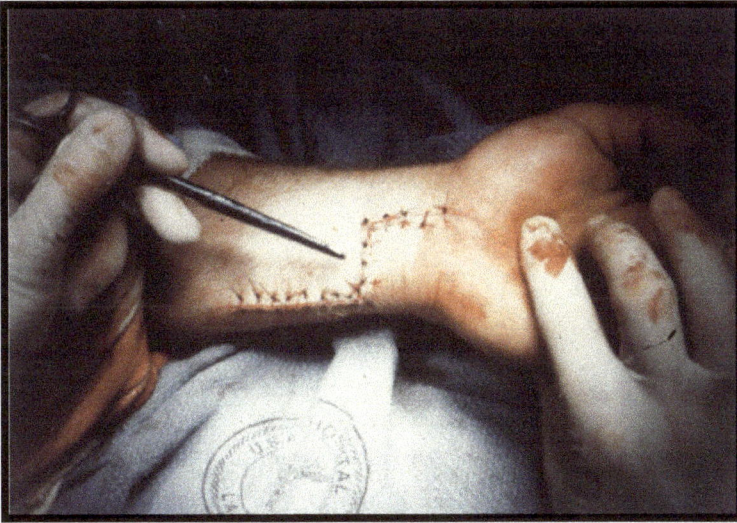

Wound closed

Now it was time to wake up the patient. The nurse anesthetist reduced the anesthetic gas slowly to lighten the patient without actually awakening him. Then, the nurse anesthetist extubated, which caused exactly what was expected: the vocal cords were stimulated causing the patient to vomit.

But we were ready. We had the patient's head turned to the side and we had suction ready to keep any stomach contents from getting into the lungs.

He vomited alcohol and peas.

Now we would have to deal with not only his surgical recovery but his alcohol withdrawal. He would need extensive physical therapy to ensure his tendons did not scar in place, which would keep him from using his hand. We also had to deal with what had been a suicide attempt, which we confirmed the next day.

There was little we could do about his relationship with his wife.

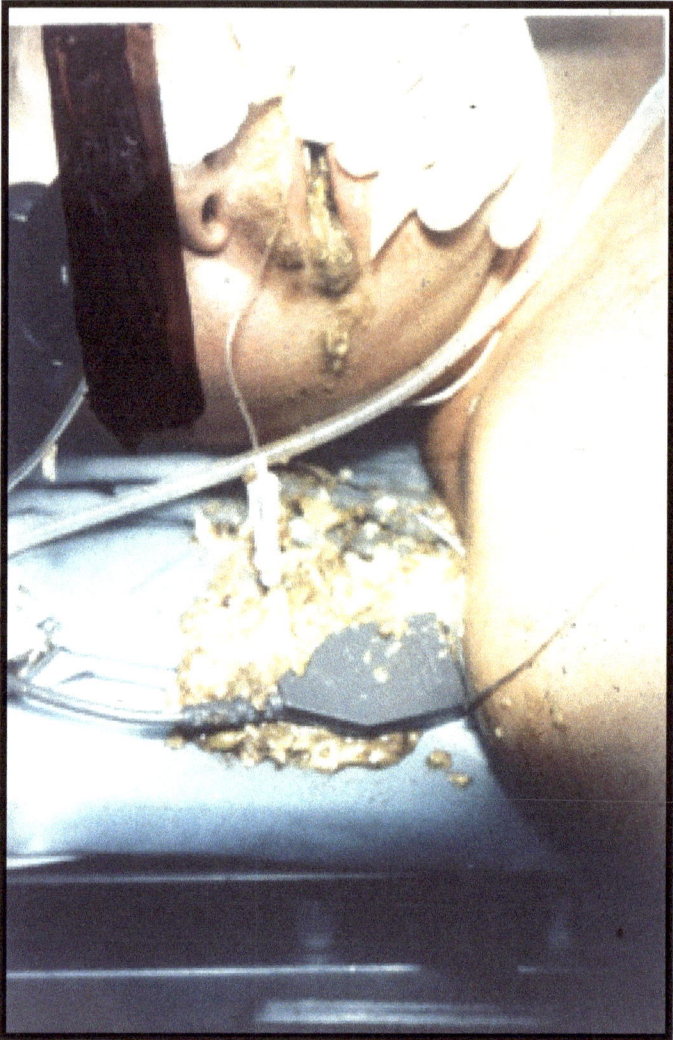

Why one must be NPO before going to the OR

Testicular Mass

It's the story for another time, place, and book, but there was a time I was assigned to cover general medical and surgical care in a remote southwestern U.S. town.

Since it was civilian care in a federal clinic, I was seeing everyone in town.

One homeless gentleman, whom I strongly suspected of being schizophrenic, would turn up in clinic at irregular intervals, asking to have his testicles removed.

Of course, I did not castrate him, despite his repeated insistence that I do so.

Then, one day, the patient came to the clinic after I had not seen him for several months.

"There's something in my testicle," he said. "You're going to have to take it off."

I examined him to find that, indeed, there was a rock-hard two-centimeter diameter mass in his right scrotal sac that appeared to be attached to his testicle. He also had palpable lymph nodes in his groin.

How did he get that large a testicular cancer since the last time I saw him? Was this a fast-growing cancer that had already spread to his lymph nodes and who knows how far beyond?

I scheduled him for the OR. He continually insisted on complete castration. I continually refused. He finally signed a consent for scrotal sac exploration, removal of scrotal mass, and possible orchiectomy (removal of the testicle) on the right side. I had no intention of getting into his left scrotal sac.

In the OR, we found a dark-colored, fibrous appearing mass surrounding his spermatic cord (containing the blood vessels to and from the testicle and the cremaster muscle that suspends the testicle) and attached to the testicle. There was no way to dissect this mass from the structures it surrounded and was attached to. We removed the mass and, with it, his right testicle.

So, he got half of his pre-op wish.

Pathology had to be sent out of town and usually took many days to return a report. I called the pathologist daily asking for the report. Finally, after what seemed like forever, the report came back.

Plant matter.

What?!

Plant matter?

Since this patient was homeless, I had no way to contact him. I was completely dependent upon his showing up in the clinic, which he did only irregularly.

When he did show up, I told him his pathology result.

"How did you get plant matter in your scrotum?" I had to ask.

"Well, Doc, since you wouldn't take my testicles off, no matter how many times I asked you to, I decided to do it myself."

"What?! How did you try?"

"I took my knife and started sawing away. But it hurt a lot and was bleeding, so I stopped."

This gentleman had one knife—an old, serrated steak knife. He used it for everything that required cutting, including his food. And he never cleaned the knife. So, when he started sawing away at his scrotum, he introduced plant matter from the knife blade into his scrotal sac.

His immune system took over, invaded the plant fibers, and cemented the foreign material to his testicle and spermatic cord.

I advised him not to try that on the other side. He didn't acknowledge my advice. I also never saw him again. You don't win them all.

Young Couple Troubles

When I was assigned to cover general medical and surgical care in a remote southwestern U.S. town, a young married couple came to see me. They were trying to conceive and were unsuccessful.

Both the husband and wife were twenty years old and had intellectual disabilities. They had met when they were institutionalized in a state facility. They stayed in the facility until they turned eighteen, when the state put them on the street. They got married and now lived in a state-subsidized apartment while receiving considerable public assistance. Either a social worker or a home health nurse visited them daily.

They both had jobs in town: he swept up the movie theater after each show, and she bagged groceries.

They wanted to speak with me about what they must be doing wrong because, try as they might, she wasn't getting pregnant.

What they didn't know was that the state, by policy, involuntarily sterilized institutionalized females when they reached menarche (first menstrual period). The state did not sterilize males. Sexist? Yes.

Side note: I have no idea if the state still has this policy.

What were my responsibilities in this case? I certainly had a responsibility to the patients in my office. Should I tell them she had been involuntarily sterilized? If I did, should I tell them that the sterilization had a good chance of being reversed surgically?

Did I have a responsibility to the state? The state, in its infinite wisdom, rendered the wife sterile to keep her from a pregnancy she had little or no mental capacity to handle.

Did I have a responsibility to an unborn child should the wife get her tubal ligation reversed? How could these two people possibly raise a child?

I didn't know what was right in this situation. I made the best decision I could at the time and didn't tell them the wife was sterilized.

I just told them to keep trying, but to realize that not everyone is successful in getting pregnant. I told them they might be one of those couples who can enjoy a life together without children.

I hope I was correct.

Ureter Scare

When I was a staff surgeon at the USAF Academy, I made it a point to visit two places every afternoon: X-ray and pathology.

Yes, in those days X-rays were on film and were read on light boxes. My philosophy was that if I ordered a film, I had better look at it myself. I am not a radiologist and do not pretend to be. But I did know my patients, and knew what I was looking for on their films.

The radiologists humored me at first, as I was the only physician of any specialty who wanted to see their own films. Everyone else was happy to read the radiologists' reports.

But, because I was there beside the radiologists every day, and was able to tell them about the patient and what I was looking for, a radiologist would see things that he had missed when he originally read the films earlier in the day.

After a while, the radiologists would wait for me to come down to read my patients' X-rays, and we would read them together. After a longer while, if one of my patient's films had been read before I got to the department, I would occasionally find things on the films the radiologists missed.

I was, and am, a firm believer in seeing any film or test that I ordered. That philosophy had stood me in good stead for as long as I was in practice. At the Air Force Academy, I oversaw Phase II Physician Assistant training. I took the PA students with me every day to read films and tried to impart that philosophy to them as well. Later, when I taught residents, I implemented the same philosophy and was very successful.

I carried that philosophy over to my pathology specimens. Anything that is removed in the operating room is sent to pathology where slides are made, read, and interpreted by the pathologist. Every day I went down to path and looked at my slides along with the pathologist. Because of my discussing the patients in person with the pathologist, my slides got second readings and, I am certain, better interpretations than the other physicians and surgeons in the hospitals where I practiced.

Now that I am done breaking my arm by patting myself on the back, I will tell you that, because I was in their department every day, I got to have a good relationship with the pathologists.

This is why I received the following phone call one late morning at the USAF Academy Hospital: "Hello, Tony, it's Phil (the pathologist). I really hate to tell you this, but I think you have made a terrible mistake in the OR."

"What?" I tried to sound calm, but I suspect I failed.

"It looks like you took out a section of ureter on one of your patients."

The previous day, I had operated on the abdomen of a retired USAF veteran and had removed a section of his anterior abdominal wall for a hernia. I was nowhere near the ureters, which are on the far posterior wall of the abdomen and behind the peritoneal cavity (the cavity that contains the small intestine and other organs).

But strange things can happen with anatomy. People have anomalies all the time. Was it possible this patient had some weird anterior ureter?

If I really cut a ureter, that meant I had cut the connection between the kidney and the bladder. And If I did that and tied it off, the kidney was backing up with urine. If I did that and didn't tie it off, it meant urine was spilling from a kidney into the peritoneal cavity.

I went down to pathology and looked at the slide with Phil. Sure enough, that specimen looked like a segment of ureter.

I had never had a complication like this, ever.

I immediately went up to the patient's bedside. With him were his wife and daughter, both of whom had made it known they hated hospitals and did not trust anything or anyone there.

I told them what the pathologist had found and tried to explain that it was not normally physically possible for me to have cut the ureter—I shouldn't have been anywhere near either one.

They weren't happy.

"What are you going to do about it?" Their question was not asked in a particularly polite fashion.

"I am ordering an IVP, which I want to send you for right now. That is an intravenous pyelogram. We put dye in your veins through your IV and the dye goes to your kidneys. The kidneys then pass the dye through your ureters into your bladder. I will be able to see if I cut a ureter or if they are both intact."

Were they happy? No. Neither was I.

Down the patient went to X-ray. I went down to read the film along with the radiologist as it came from the processor.

Low and behold, both kidneys, both ureters, and the urinary bladder were intact and completely normal.

Thank goodness!

Before I went back to the patient's room to tell him and his family, I went to see Phil.

"Phil, the ureters on my patient are completely intact."

"Oh," he calmly said. "I guess he must have had a *patent urachus*. Sorry about that."

The urachus is a fetal structure that looks like a ureter under the microscope. Normally it is found on the anterior abdominal wall, and normally it closes after a baby is born. But having one stay open, or patent, is considered a normal anatomical variant.

Suppressing the urge to strangle Phil, I left pathology and explained all of this to the patient and his fuming family. I think they may have already contacted a lawyer. I hated disappointing them.

Breast Cancer with a Surprise

One of the family practitioners sent me a pleasant but very worried sixty-two-year-old woman for a palpable breast mass.

With her husband in the examining room, I did a breast exam and easily found the mass. I suspected it was fibrocystic, which is a commonly found benign condition.

During the exam the patient stated, "I've never had a mammogram."

One of the great things about military medicine was how rapidly we could get needed studies. I sent her and her husband down to radiology, she scheduled her mammogram, and I saw her back the next week with the X-rays in hand.

The palpable mass did not appear suspicious for cancer on the mammogram—it looked like what we expect with benign fibrocystic changes. However, deep in the breast was another finding: a cluster of microcalcifications that looked suspicious for cancer.

Later that week, I did a needle-localized breast biopsy.

Four days later, she and her husband were back in my office when I gave them the results: infiltrating ductal carcinoma.

We had a long discussion resulting in the patient requesting a mastectomy. But she also wanted immediate reconstruction.

My first assistant on the mastectomy was one of the Air Force Academy Hospital's plastic and reconstructive surgeons. After completing the mastectomy, we changed gowns, gloves, and instruments, and re-prepped and re-draped the patient. The reconstructive guy and I changed sides of the OR table so he could take over as primary surgeon with me as his first assistant.

Together we performed a TRAM flap. TRAM stands for Transverse Rectus Abdominis Myocutaneous flap reconstruction.

To do a TRAM, an incision is made in the abdomen and a segment of the rectus abdominis muscle—also known as the "six pack" muscle—is removed with its overlying abdominal fat. The muscle and fat are tunneled under the abdominal and chest skin to the area of the breast, accompanied by the blood supply to the muscle. A TRAM flap provides the patient with a natural appearing breast when she is in her clothes.

Post-operatively, the patient had an uneventful recovery. After an appropriate surgical follow-up, I returned the patient to her family physician. She no longer needed a surgeon, so, unless she had a new surgical problem, I did not expect to see her again until her six-month follow-up appointment.

A few weeks before the scheduled six-month follow-up, I was walking down the hallway of the USAF Hospital heading for my clinic. There, sitting outside my office were the patient and her husband, looking worried and clutching each other's hand. As soon as she saw me, she exclaimed, "Doctor, the cancer is back in the new breast you gave me!"

I turned to the sergeant running the clinic and asked him to hold the other patients waiting to be seen, then took the patient and her husband into my exam room.

I was expecting to see a cutaneous metastasis, as I could not think what else would make the patient think there was cancer in the TRAM flap. But there was nothing to be seen, or felt, on the examination.

"I'm not seeing or feeling anything. Please tell me what causes you to think there is cancer in the flap?"

"My new breast is getting bigger!"

I tried to reassure her and her husband that her flap getting bigger was not normally a sign of cancer, especially as this was not actually breast tissue. But to be complete and help the patient's peace of mind I picked up the phone and called radiology.

"Will you please do an immediate mammogram on the patient I am sending down to you, have the radiologist read it, and send her back to me with the films?"

Off she and her husband went to radiology. I saw my scheduled clinic patients until she and her husband came back carrying the films. Which were, as expected, completely negative.

"What has changed in your life since the last time I saw you?" I asked.

The patient's husband told me that since the surgery, she had fallen in love with doughnuts.

"That explains it," I said. "Remember your new breast is not really a breast. It's abdominal fat that has been moved to your chest. If your diet would cause an increase in the fat of your abdomen, that will also make this 'breast' abdominal fat increase in size."

"I always wanted to be a little bigger upstairs," she said. "I guess I never expected it to happen this way!"

Mystery Injury

The Azores are islands in the middle of the Atlantic Ocean about 900-or-so miles west of Portugal. My family and I spent two years there.

The U.S. Air Force hospital at that time had seven beds and a four-bed "close observation unit." We called it "close observation" as we didn't have an ICU. We had six doctors: three family physicians, an obstetrician/gynecologist, a pediatrician, and me as the general surgeon. We had a nurse anesthetist for anesthesia. If we wanted X-rays, we had two X-ray techs but we read our own films. No CT. No MRI (hadn't been invented yet). No ultrasound. We did have a lab that could do basic lab work. Our wartime mission was to expand to forty beds after receiving more staff.

We had an ER that had to be staffed 24/7, but, as I said, only six doctors. So, we took turns covering the ER for 24 hours at a time in addition to our regular duties. Because I was also the Chief of Hospital Services, I made the ER schedule. I always covered it on Sundays from 7 am until 7 am Monday so the other doctors could have a weekend day off with their families.

One Sunday, right at 7 a.m, the ER called me to say I needed to get there ASAP from the on-call room. I asked what the matter was. The tech told me to just please get there.

That is a scary thing to be told. Our ER techs were excellent people, all well-trained and experienced. So, to be told, "Just get here," could mean anything, but none of the options were good.

I quickly walked to the ER to find a twenty-one-year-old active-duty airman sitting on a gurney, wearing a hospital gown, accompanied by his twenty-year-old wife. Both the airman and his wife looked very frightened.

I asked, "What is the problem?"

The ER tech silently lifted the patient's gown and showed me the patient's penis.

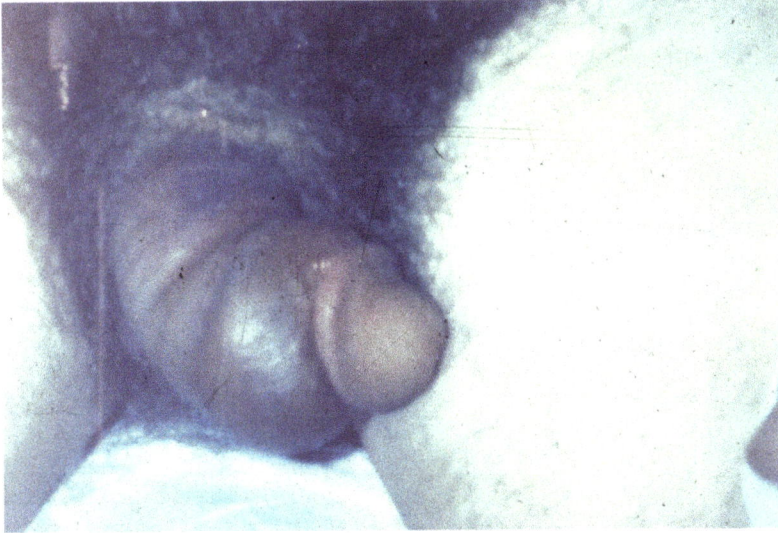

Swollen, blood-filled, deformed penis

His penis was filled with blood and bent at a ninety-degree angle pointing to the left.

"How did this happen?" I asked.

"I had an erection and rolled over in bed."

Hmmm....

I said, "I've had erections and rolled over in bed, and this has never happened to me. So, what really happened?"

"I had an erection and rolled over in bed."

Since I knew that could not possibly be the cause of this injury, I took the wife out into the hallway and asked her what really happened. This was not morbid curiosity on my part. One usually decides how to treat surgical injuries based on what is called the "mechanism of injury." If you know how an injury happened, you can more easily assess what other injuries might be consequential. This helps you formulate a plan for treatment.

The wife stared at me—clearly frightened and conflicted—hesitated a moment, then said, "He had an erection and rolled over in bed."

Now I knew that they had rehearsed the story on the way to the ER. I further knew I was not going to get a true mechanism of injury from either of them.

Truthfully, I did not know what to do for this patient. In my residency, I had studied no urology at all. So, I called Andrews Air Force Base in Washington, D.C., woke the on-call urologist, and described what I was seeing.

The urologist said, "Sounds like a fractured penis."

I had never heard of a fractured penis.

"So, what do I do for it?" I asked.

He said, "Send the patient to radiology for a *corpus cavernosum* study."

I reminded him that I was calling from the Azores. We didn't have a radiology department. We didn't have a radiologist. I told him if I wanted any kind of study, I had to get it myself. And I didn't know how to do a corpus cavernosum study.

The corpus cavernosum (plural is corpora cavernosa) are two tubes of very tough connective tissue in the penis (and clitoris) that fill with blood to give people erections. The urologist was telling me this patient may have fractured—in essence, torn—the connective tissue of one of his corpora cavernosa.

He asked me if I had any water-soluble dye, and I told him I did. He said to get a syringe of dye and inject it into the corpus cavernosum that the penis is pointing toward. If I could fill that corpus fully, veins that connect the two corpora cavernosa would push dye into the other corpus. If that corpus was fractured, the dye would leak out and under the skin around the fractured corpus. He then said to put an X-ray plate under the penis and shoot a film. If there was a fracture, I would see the extravasated dye and could make the diagnosis.

I thanked the guy, apologized for waking him, and did exactly what he suggested. Sure enough, the right corpus cavernosum was fractured.

I then called the urologist back and re-awakened him.

"Yup, he has a fractured corpus cavernosum," I said. "What do you want me to do about it?"

He said, "How fast can you get the patient to Andrews?"

"Well, let's see. A minimum of forty-eight hours to get a MedEvac plane here, assuming the weather permits. Then travel time. So, at the very least, sixty hours."

"That's too long," he said. "If you want this guy to get erections for the rest of his life, you will need to operate on him and fix the corpus."

"OK," said I. "But I have never seen that operation, much less done one in the past. I don't even have a surgical atlas of urologic surgeries to look at."

Remember, this was before the internet.

"No problem," he said. "Just make a circumferential incision at the base of the glans (tip) of the penis and skeletonize the penis. Be careful of the lateral nerves, or he'll never get another erection. Then sew up the tear, close the skin, and you're done."

Skeletonize means to dissect the overlying skin from the underlying structures in the penis.

With trepidation, I took the patient to the OR. I called the OB/GYN doctor to assist me, as she was the only other person on the island with surgical experience.

You should have heard her when I told her what I was asking her to help me with. "We're going to do what??"

So, the nurse-anesthetist put the patient to sleep, and I made a circumferential incision at the base of the glans penis.

There, covered in clotted blood, was a fractured corpus cavernosum.

After cleaning off the blood clot, the tear was an "L" shape that looked like this:

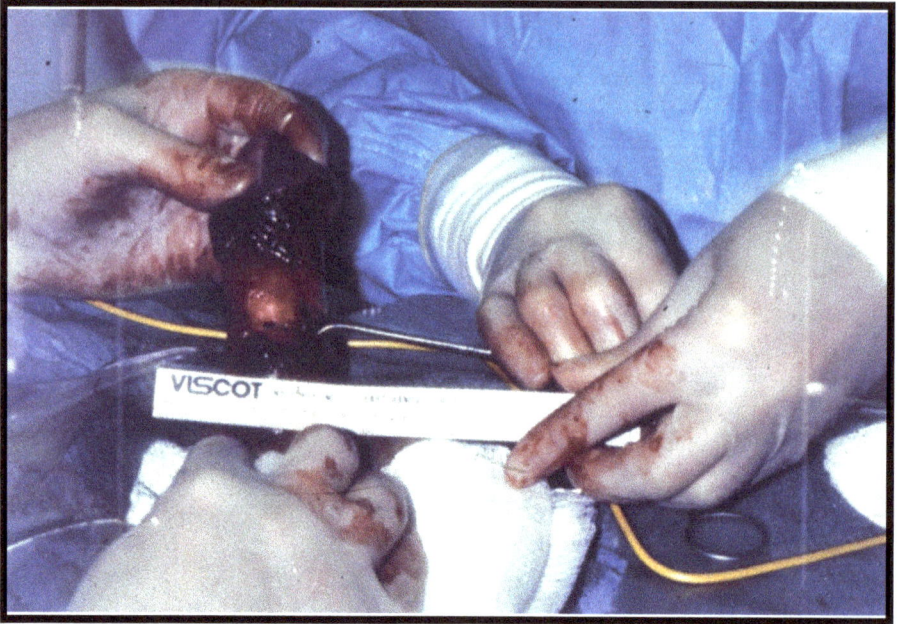

Initial exposure of blood-covered corpus cavernosum

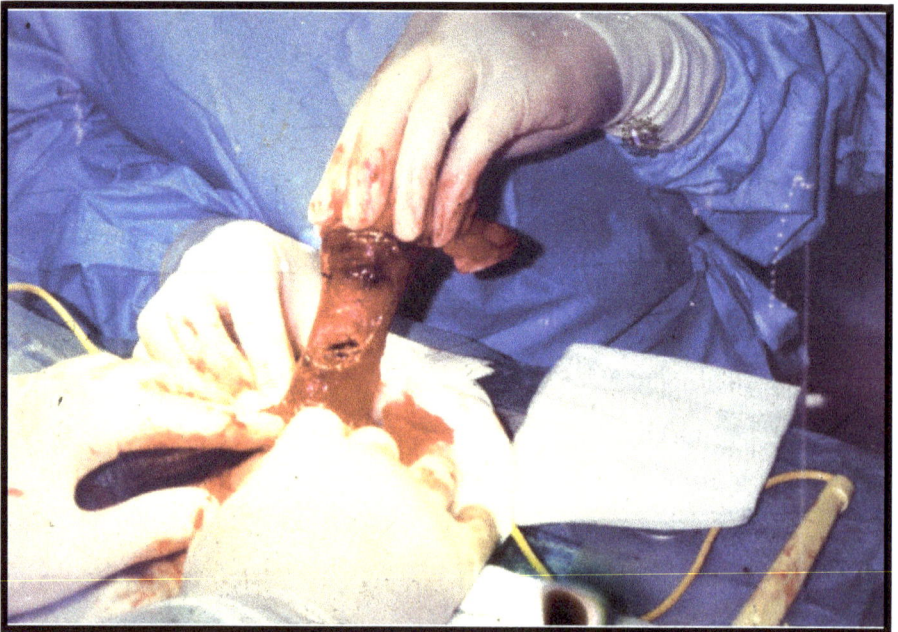

Corpus cavernosal laceration after cleaning away the blood

Now I had the problem of figuring out how to repair the connective tissue wall of the corpus cavernosum. Because of the way the blood supply to the penis works, men get regular erections in the night, usually up to seven or so. I didn't want to repair his penis only to have the stitches tear out when he got an erection.

Also, the skin overlying the penis is tissue-paper thin. Any sutures I put in the corpus would be felt through the skin, especially the knots.

I discounted using a non-absorbable suture because of the thinness of the skin. I felt the knots would poke through the skin. The usual stitches one uses on tissue such as that of the penis would dissolve too quickly. I settled on a woven, dissolvable suture that would be gone in a few weeks and hoped that was the correct decision.

Then I closed the skin.

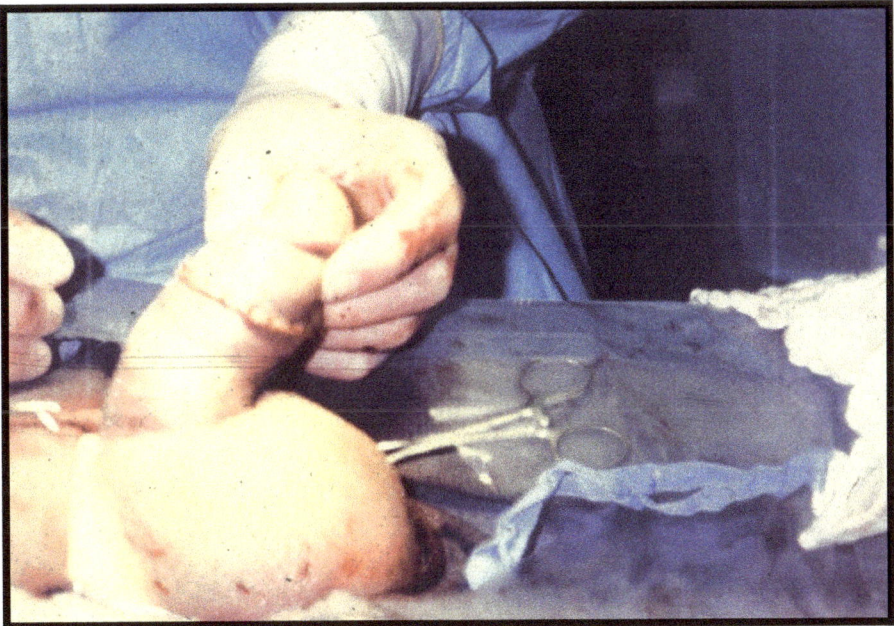

Penile closure

Now I got to worrying about those erections that men get at night. I figured no one would get an erection if he had a foley catheter in, so I asked for the largest diameter foley we had. This thing was a monster. I put it in, and we woke him up.

I then called for a MedEvac plane, and, about sixty hours later, the patient and his wife were at Andrews Air Force Base in Washington, D.C.

A couple of weeks later who should be sitting in my clinic but the airman and his wife. I called them into an exam room, and they sat side-by-side, holding hands.

"How did it go in D.C.?" I asked.

"It went fine. They told me you fixed me up fine. Thanks, Doc. But they said I didn't need that foley."

They thought you didn't need the foley, but I did.

By this time I had gotten a book flown in (remember, internet not yet invented) and looked up penile fractures. I now knew the most likely causes, none of which involved getting an erection and rolling over in bed because that cannot cause a penile fracture.

I then asked, "So tell me, what really happened to cause this?"

Holding hands, they visibly squeezed them more tightly, turned to look at each other, then looked at me.

"I had an erection and rolled over in bed."

Side note: A couple of days after I sent the patient and his wife off to D.C., and before they returned, I was sitting in my Chief of Hospital Services Office doing paperwork when I was paged overhead to come to the ER stat. I walked quickly to the ER to find the entire medical staff (five other doctors), most of the nurses, and a significant number of the other staff standing in the ER.

I didn't see a patient on a gurney.

Yet I had been paged stat.

"What's up?" I asked.

One of the family practice doctors said, "We have an X-ray we need you to look at." He pointed to a view box on the ER wall.

There was an X-ray of a penis. In the center of the penis was a bone. The bone was fractured.

"Looks like a fractured penis," I said while the entire room laughed.

Of course, a real human penis does not have a bone in it. What these comedians had done was get a chicken femur, fracture it, then place the fractured bone in a Playdoh® penis and get an X-ray.

I wish I had that X-ray now. It was a classic!

For the two years I was assigned to the Air Force Academy Hospital I was on call either every third or every fourth night. It seemed there was someone with appendicitis virtually every single night I was on call.

When I got orders to transfer from the Air Force Academy Hospital, the OR crew gave me an award. The inscription says, *"Order of the Appy Award. He Didn't Leave an Appendix in Colorado Springs."*

The knife handle says, "A Little Slice of Heaven." After each case, no matter how the case went, I always said to the OR crew, "Thanks everyone. It was a little slice of heaven." I guess they were listening.

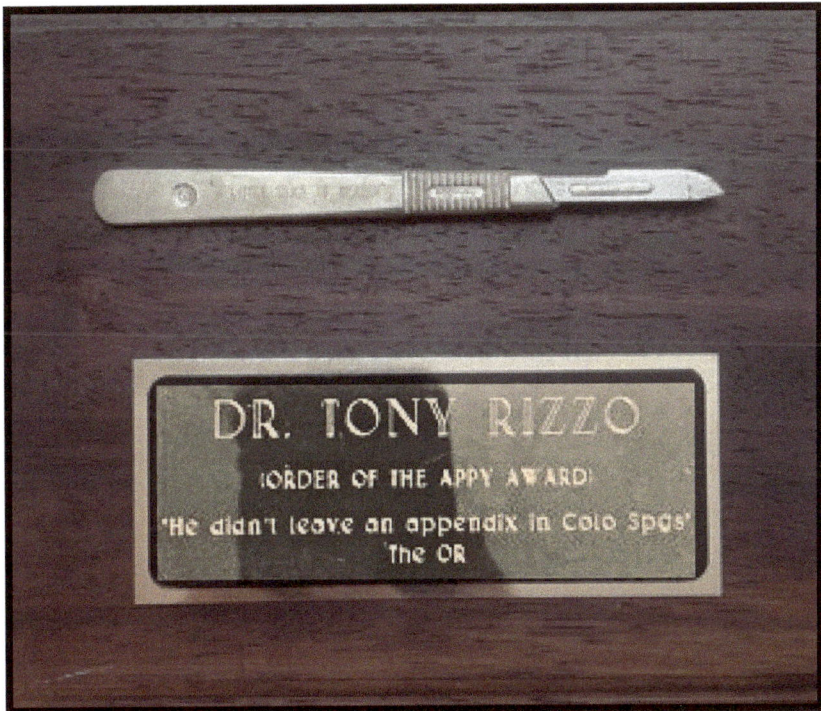

Order of the Appy Award

Teaching Attending

An Unexpected Transition

I left Air Force active duty to teach surgery in a civilian family practice residency. But I loved the Air Force and had planned to make it a career. Here's what happened:

While on active duty I was writing a book about Disney stuff—my family was (and is) a Disney family. During my book research I found out about a Disney project called Celebration. After making a number of phone calls I got in touch with the Celebration project manager. I explained who I was and told him about my book. He invited me to come to Orlando for a meeting.

I immediately asked for a one-week leave (what the military calls a vacation) and took my family to Walt Disney World. While they were in the parks I met with the Celebration project manager. He explained that Celebration was to be a new town on Disney property that was in the planning stages. That meeting led to him requesting my input about various plans for Celebration. He sent me a series of questions to which I responded with lengthy answers—sometimes twenty-page answers to a single question.

A few weeks later, at the Air Force Academy, I got a phone call from the Celebration project manager. He stated he wanted me to come to Orlando and be on the team to plan the Celebration hospital. Disney had already contracted with a local medical center group (let's call them Medical Center A) to plan the hospital. Medical Center A had a family practice residency. The project manager stated he had arranged for me to apply to become a full-time faculty member in the residency, teaching surgery, and that I would contribute to planning the hospital while teaching. He even said he could guarantee a lot in Celebration on which I could build a house (later reneged on).

I flew to Orlando, had a cursory interview with Medical Center A's residency director, and was offered the job.

I thought this was my retirement dream being handed to me. I had planned on a twenty-year career in the USAF, then wanted to find a residency in or near Orlando that would let me teach surgery while having my family live near Walt Disney World. I was only nine years towards my Air Force twenty years, so taking the offered job would mean leaving the Air Force and losing my retirement investment.

But there was a way to take the job and stay in the Air Force! The Guard and Reserves! It didn't take long to find a USAF Guard, then Reserve unit near Orlando, both of which were happy to have me. I could continue to serve, continue toward my eventual USAF retirement, teach surgery in a civilian residency, and be part of a new town on Disney property.

I couldn't turn it down.

Helicopters

Although I didn't perform surgery on either of the next two patients, I am including them to demonstrate the stark contrast between how the U.S. military and our allies operate.

One afternoon at Patrick Air Force Base in Cocoa Beach, Florida, we received an emergency request for assistance from a US Navy destroyer at sea. I was commanding an Aeromedical Staging Squadron in the USAF Reserve and flew, as a flight surgeon, with a rscue squadron. this was when I also taught surgery in Medical Center A, described below. It was the end of the duty day, and every crew member had flown that day. Thus, launching a mission required a written waiver from the wing commander.

"Is this a life-threatening emergency, Doc?"

"Yes, Sir, it is," I answered. "The message is that a sailor has fallen down a well connecting decks on the destroyer, landing on his head. The corpsman aboard believes the man has a broken neck."

The wing king signed a waiver. The crews quickly planned an emergency mission.

Two HH-60 air-refuelable helicopters would launch with a C-130 air refueler. Given the distance to the destroyer, both helicopters would have to air refuel multiple times to complete the mission.

I was on helicopter one, which was the primary rescue helicopter. The second helicopter was launched with a parajumper medic as our backup should we go down or have to abort for any reason.

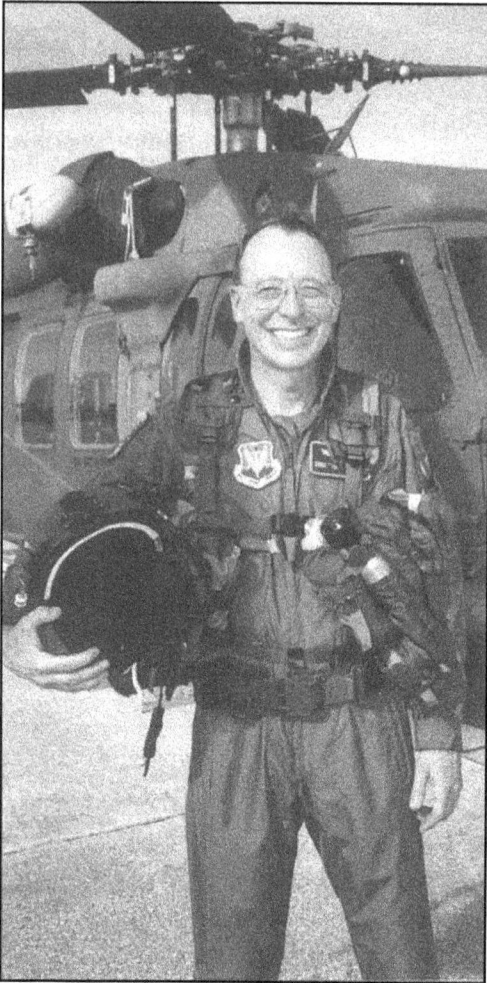

Standing in front of the HH-60 Helicopter

It was after dark when we launched into severe weather. The winds were blowing at forty knots, and the seas had twenty-foot waves. It was very turbulent. We had removed the seats from the back of the helicopter to allow us to bring a stretcher aboard.

The entire mission was performed using night vision goggles. We were each wearing twenty pounds of gear, including the five-and-a-quarter-pound helmet/night vision goggle combination.

We flew for three turbulent hours to get to the ship. During that time, we air-refueled three times, the third time just as we got to the destroyer.

The initial plan was to land on the destroyer. This was not a good plan. The ship had turned on every light it could to guide us to it. But we were wearing night vision goggles. All that light flared our goggles, blinding us.

Our pilot asked the ship to turn off all its lights except the red light on the tip of the mast. Now we could see fine—night vision goggles work well—but the sailors aboard the ship were in the dark.

Air Force pilots are amazingly talented people. But they are not trained to land on a destroyer that is pitching and rolling in twenty-foot seas while fighting a forty-knot wind. So, Plan Number One, landing on the destroyer, went out the window.

Plan Number Two was to lower me to the ship. Another stupid idea.

I struggled into a "poopie suit" in addition to my other gear. A poopie suit is a rubber, one-piece garment that goes over all your equipment except for your LPU—Life Preserver Unit. The suit has tight closures around the neck, wrists, and ankles. It is designed to be waterproof and to float, as well as preserve body heat should I fall into the ocean. It looked like there was a decent chance I would fall into the ocean and have to survive until daybreak when people could look for me.

We had a jungle penetrator that we attached to the winch out of the starboard side of the helicopter. A jungle penetrator is a heavy metal apparatus that looks like a big bullet. I jumped out of the helicopter, caught the jungle penetrator, and strapped myself to it.

The flight engineer started to lower me as the pilot tried to hover over the stern of the destroyer. The pilot hovered by keeping the ship's mast light directly in front of him. The helicopter pitched and rolled as the pilot kept station with the pitching, rolling masthead. I swung like a giant pendulum over the ship.

It was clear to me that, if the jungle penetrator actually encountered the ship, I would be crushed. I was glad that fact became apparent to the helicopter crew, as I had no communication with them. All I could see was the ship wildly passing below me, back and forth, up and down, side to side, as I swung crazily above the ship. It was black—green—black—green—black, which was the black water on either side of the ship and the green ship flashing by—green because I was seeing it using night vision.

After I had been swinging like that for quite a while, the flight engineer winched me back into the helicopter, and I plugged my helmet into the comms to talk with the crew. Clearly, neither landing nor lowering me was going to work.

So, we tried Plan Number Three. The engineer threw a light line with a weight on the end onto the destroyer. The words in that sentence do not do justice to how difficult that was to accomplish. The forty-knot winds, our main rotor downwash, and the ship's constant movement in relation to the helicopter meant the line was thrown many, many, many times before it hit the destroyer and was picked up by a crewman.

A crewman tied a heavier line to the end of our line, and the engineer hoisted the heavier line up to the helicopter. Next, the engineer untied our light line from the ship's line and attached the end of our metal winch line. The crew could then pull our winch line onto the destroyer as the engineer let out the line.

All the while, the pilots were struggling to keep us hovering more or less over the stern of the rolling, pitching ship.

With our winch line now on the deck, the Navy crewmen brought the injured man to the deck. Once the Stokes stretcher was attached to our winch line, the flight engineer started to raise the injured man. Immediately, the stretcher began to rotate and swing wildly.

The injured man was strapped to the stretcher and completely immobilized. He could not see, as it was a pitch-black night. He had no control and no way to help himself as he was blasted by our rotor wash and the forty-knot winds. It had to be terrifying to be in the stretcher, swinging and spinning and blasted by wind.

But we finally got him aboard the helicopter. The flight engineer helped me get an IV going and begin care for the sailor as we headed for shore and a hospital.

We had air refueled as we reached the destroyer. We were at bingo fuel (almost empty) when he got the injured man aboard. We immediately hit the C-130 tanker.

We then started for the nearest shore, which turned out to be Camp Lejune in North Carolina. It was still far enough away that we had to air refuel a fifth time before arriving.

We landed at the Naval Hospital at Camp Lejune. The ER waiting room was filled with retirees and dependents when we came through the doors in full gear and with a clearly critical patient. I could see the looks on the faces of the people who were waiting to be seen—they immediately knew their wait was going to be longer now that this patient had arrived.

Contrast the above mission with a helicopter rescue from when I was on active duty in the Azores:

One morning we received a call for an injured U.S. Navy sailor aboard a destroyer who needed immediate care. In the Azores the only helicopters belonged to the Portuguese Air Force.

The Portuguese helicopters did not have the ability to air refuel.

But the Portuguese said they would be more than willing to fly way beyond the range of their helicopters to rescue the Navy crewman if I went with them. They wanted me because they did not have a flight doctor or a corpsman who could go to care for the patient on the way back to the hospital.

I said I would go but asked how they planned to air refuel.

"Don't worry about it!" they said.

I grabbed a med bag and went down to the flightline to find two helicopters and crews ready to go. Unlike the helicopter rescue I already described, the weather was clear with little wind and no storms.

I looked in the back of the helicopter and found the area for the patient was filled with five-gallon gas cans.

I had no headset and did not speak Portuguese, so it was a long ride in silence while I worried about running out of fuel over the Atlantic Ocean.

I need not have been concerned.

All the way out to the destroyer, the engineer intermittently pulled up a floorboard and exposed an access hatch to a fuel tank. He would then pour fuel from a can into the tank, throw the gas can out of the helicopter's door into the ocean, look at me, and grin.

By the time we got to the destroyer, he had thrown out so many cans that there was plenty of room for the stretcher, which we hoisted aboard with a winch.

Much lower tech than our HH-60s and C-130s. But it worked just fine.

Acute Abdominal Pain

I was teaching surgery to family practice residents. Essentially, I was the entire surgery service in the residency. First year (intern) FP residents rotated for three months at a time with me.

One evening, the ER paged surgery for a forty-year-old man with severe abdominal pain. The intern saw him and immediately called me in.

When I saw the patient, he was in acute distress with severe abdominal pain and a board-rigid abdomen. A board-rigid abdomen means the abdominal muscles are in spasm to try to keep the abdomen from moving. This happens when an intra-abdominal catastrophe has occurred, stimulating the lining of the abdominal cavity called the peritoneum. The peritoneum is exquisitely innervated for pain, and when the spinal nerves to the peritoneum are stimulated, the overlying abdominal muscles, also innervated by the same spinal nerves, go into spasm.

The patient was in shock with falling blood pressure and rapid pulse and fever.

Given the severity of his condition, there was no time to get studies to try to diagnose what might have happened in his abdomen. His only chance for survival was exploratory laparotomy. Basically, we would cut him open and look around to find the problem, then try to fix it.

I sent off basic labs, but there was no time to get back the results. The patient was deteriorating that quickly.

I asked the patient if he had any illnesses for which he was receiving medical treatment. He vigorously denied all past medical history. He stated he had no illnesses and was on no medications.

Further, he emphatically asked—even begged—for me to do anything and everything possible to save his life.

I asked him if he had family with him. He stated he was all alone with no family in the world.

He signed a surgical consent for exploratory laparotomy and repair of whatever we might find in his abdomen that was clearly killing him. The consent included all post-operative care, to include being on a ventilator and getting intensive care.

When the intern and I made a midline incision in the patient's abdomen several liters of pus, blood, and stool rolled out of his abdomen, soaking my gown and my underlying scrub pants and socks and filling my shoes.

After evacuating his abdominal cavity, we discovered he had a perforated colon. Spontaneously perforating the colon is not something that occurs easily or without some underlying pathology.

We resected the perforated colon and created a colostomy. Anesthesia was quite busy resuscitating this extremely sick man. We closed him up and wheeled him to the recovery room on a ventilator and multiple intravenous antibiotics and antifungals. His next stop was going to be the intensive care unit.

He was in septic shock, had had a major surgery, and was looking at, at best, a fifty-fifty chance of recovery. Septic shock is the leading cause of death in ICUs in the United States. It has a forty-percent mortality, and that mortality goes up fifteen percent for every system that fails. This patient had a perforated colon and was on a ventilator, so, as I said, his chances were less than fifty-fifty.

While I was sitting in the recovery room writing his post-op orders, a nurse told me the patient's next of kin wanted to see me.

The patient had specifically stated he did not have any next of kin.

Puzzled, I asked the nurse to bring this supposed next of kin back.

In walked a young man who stated he was the patient's companion. Those were the days when gay marriage was not recognized. Today, the man would likely have been the patient's husband. But then, the man I was speaking with had no legal authority or rights.

The companion stated the patient had AIDS and was receiving multiple medications to treat the illness. This information was completely at odds with what the patient had told us pre-op, but it was not unusual at the time when having HIV/AIDS was a stigmatized condition.

Further, the partner said the patient had a living will instructing that the patient was not to receive surgery of any kind, was never to be intubated, was never to get IVs, and was never to be admitted to an ICU.

The companion insisted that we follow the living will.

I explained that the patient had signed a consent that was diametrically opposite to what the living will stated.

While there is now case law that states a living will can be reversed by a current, signed consent, that case law had not yet been tried when I saw this patient.

I called the hospital administrator on call and explained the entire situation. The administrator told me to follow the living will (again, today that would not be the case).

That meant turning off the ventilator and stopping the IVs.

Within minutes of doing so, I pronounced the patient dead.

These were the early days of HIV and AIDS in the United States. Much was not known about the virus or how it could be spread other than by blood-to-blood contact. Treatments were primitive. Preventive measures were guesswork.

I mention this because I had a rash on my ankle that I had scratched in the surgical changing room while putting on my scrubs for this operation. I had scratched the rash to the point that it had bled.

I had then stood, soaked in this patient's blood, pus, and stool for two hours while trying to save his life.

Now the patient was dead.

I called one of the internal medicine attendings with whom I taught the residents and explained what had happened.

He stated he had no idea if I could get HIV and thus AIDS by soaking my bloody rash in infected body fluids for two hours, but he was certainly worried that I could. He started me on the most effective antiviral HIV medication that was known at the time and suggested I take it for six months. Then I could be tested to see if I had gotten HIV.

I was terrified. I had a wife and young children. If I got AIDS from this patient, my family would be left with little or nothing. At that point, I had only a life insurance policy with which to support my family if I was gone.

For six months I was afraid to kiss or even touch my wife and children. The medication gave me an unremitting, massively severe headache and sensitivity to light. But I had to keep seeing patients, teaching residents, and operating, as that was how I supported my family.

Fortunately, after six months my HIV test was negative. We tentatively stopped the antivirals and tested again in six months. Negative.

Subsequently, I had yearly tests for the next two decades. All negative. Thank goodness.

More Abdominal Pain

One noon, at the hospital where I was teaching residents, a sixty-eight-year-old woman presented to the ER complaining of severe abdominal pain.

The ER was exceptionally busy.

The triage nurse noted that the patient's vital signs were all normal. The patient did not have a fever, and had a normal pulse, blood pressure, and respirations. So, without checking with anyone, the nurse put the patient in the back hall to await a time when the emergency medicine resident would be able to examine her.

The patient was not checked by anyone for the four hours she spent lying on a gurney in the back hall.

At the four-hour mark, the emergency medicine resident saw the patient. He noted her abdomen was tender to palpation with rebound. Rebound is when the examiner presses on an abdomen and quickly removes his or her hand. This rapid motion shakes the peritoneum (covering of the abdominal organs) and, if there is tenderness with rapidly removing the hand it signifies peritonitis. Peritonitis is inflammation of the lining of the abdominal cavity and is usually a sign of an intra-abdominal problem—or a catastrophe.

Vital signs were not repeated. The resident noted the four-hour-old normal vital signs and decided the patient was not urgently ill.

The resident paged my resident, who was a family practice intern rotating on surgery.

My intern was busy on the ward, so he asked the ER resident if this was an urgent emergency. Based on the four-hour-old normal vital signs, the ER resident said it was not.

So, another full hour went by before my intern went down to the ER to evaluate the patient. Being an intern, and not one who was planning a career in surgery, he was not yet very good at his job. But he was smart and thoughtful. He ordered labs and both abdominal and chest X-rays.

All of that took more time.

The labs and X-rays came back, but the intern did not know how to read the films. The radiologist was taking call from home, so no one saw the films except for the intern.

Finally, at 7:00 p.m., the intern called me. I was just finishing dinner at home.

The intern said he had a patient with abdominal pain, an increased white blood cell count, with a left shift (indicative of infection), and X-rays of the chest and abdomen he was quite sure were abnormal but that he really didn't know how to interpret.

"What are her vital signs?" I asked.

"The only vital signs were taken at noon, and they were normal."

"You're telling me someone with abdominal pain has been in the ER for seven hours and has only had arrival vital signs?"

The intern hesitated. He immediately knew he should have noticed that deficiency in the patient's care. "That's right," he admitted.

"I'm on my way," I said.

I got to the ER at 7:30. The first thing I did after introducing myself to the patient was get a set of vital signs. The patient had a fever, her blood pressure was 90/40, her pulse was 100, and her respirations were twenty-five. She was in shock.

Her abdomen was board-rigid from guarding—the spinal nerves to her abdominal organs putting her abdominal muscles into spasm—a sure sign of an intra-abdominal crisis.

The intern, now clearly worried that he had missed a serious problem, asked me about the X-rays.

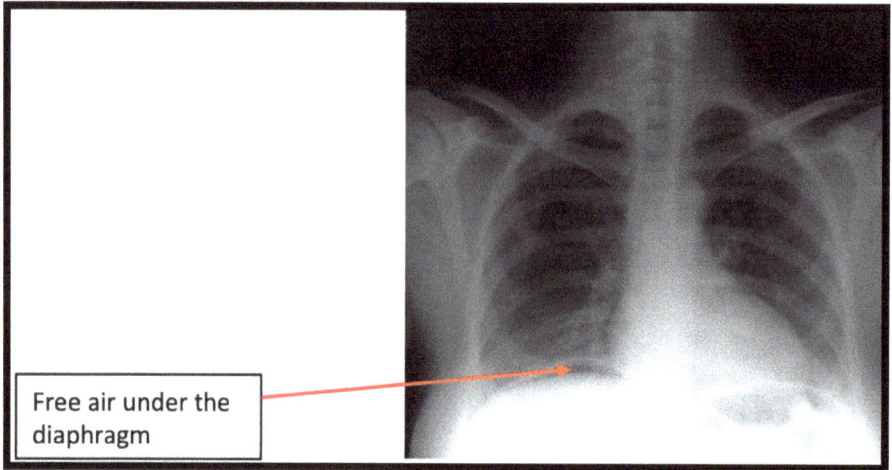

Free air under the diaphragm

Free Air Under the Diaphragm

"That's free air under the diaphragm—air between the liver and the diaphragm. There's not supposed to be air in the abdominal cavity at all. So start telling me all the organs that can contain gas," I said.

"Uh, the stomach; the colon; I think that's it."

"Normally you're correct. But anywhere there are bacteria there can be gas, so include the small intestine."

"So, what does it mean?" he asked me.

"It means something that normally contains gas has ruptured or been perforated, leaking the gas out into the peritoneal cavity (abdominal cavity). Gas rises. So, when she sat up for the upright chest X-ray, the free gas in her peritoneal cavity rose and collected between the liver and diaphragm. This is definitely on the bad list."

Tongue in cheek, I frequently talked to my residents about a "good list" and a "bad list" of things that happen to patients. This most definitely was high on the bad list.

The patient's serum amylase came back from the lab, and it was elevated. Now I knew with confidence that she had perforated a gastric (stomach) ulcer. I could surmise the perforation was on the posterior aspect (back wall) of the stomach and that gastric acid had leaked out of the stomach and was burning into the pancreas. The pancreas sits behind the stomach.

A hole in the stomach would release gas into the peritoneal cavity, resulting in the free air under the diaphragm seen on chest X-ray. The inflammation of her pancreas would explain her pain. Infection with organisms leaking from the stomach would give her sepsis, resulting in the shock she was experiencing.

This was serious.

The patient was now moving in and out of consciousness. When she was conscious, I rapidly explained what was going on and obtained consent for surgery.

I asked her if she had any relatives we could call. She stated her "close friend" was in the waiting room. This was long before society openly accepted gay relationships, and the idea of gay marriage was most definitely not in anyone's mind.

Nonetheless, I understood that homosexuality was biologically innate and was not a "choice." Although she had no legal standing at the time, I had the ER staff bring the "close friend" back. I explained everything to the friend who said she wanted everything possible done to save the patient's life.

The patient had signed a consent for surgery. The friend wanted everything done. It's important to keep that in mind.

In the OR, we found a perforated gastric ulcer on the posterior wall of the stomach. We oversewed the ulcer, irrigated the abdomen to try to mitigate the diffuse peritonitis we found, put in drains, started broad-spectrum antibiotics and antifungals, and closed her up.

In the recovery room, the patient was clearly still in shock—as expected. She was intubated and on a ventilator. Given her septic shock condition and the diffuse nature of her peritonitis she was looking at a prolonged ICU stay. I've mentioned before that sepsis is the number one cause of death in ICUs in the United States. This patient was far from being out of the woods. There was a good chance she would die.

I explained all of this to the friend in the recovery room.

The friend replied that the patient did not have a living will, but that the patient "always said she did not want to be on machines—if I have to be on a breathing machine let me go."

The patient was on a ventilator and would continue to be—possibly for weeks.

The patient had signed surgical consent. Did that mean she understood she might come out of the OR on a ventilator? Possibly not.

The friend had no legal status. But the friend, who had wanted everything possible done for the patient, now insisted we turn everything off and let the patient die.

I called the hospital administrator on call and explained the entire situation. The hospital administrator told me we should do everything humanly possible to save this patient because he was worried about the hospital being sued. He clearly understood that the seven-and-one-half-hour delay in initiating treatment, the delay in the ER doctor seeing the patient, the absence of regular vital signs being obtained, and the mistriage by the ER nurse, all likely contributed to the patient's current critical condition. The administrator wanted the hospital protected, and he saw saving this patient as the only route to that end.

I had a long, sit-down talk with the friend, who, as I said, should have been considered the patient's spouse. The friend was horribly conflicted. She loved the patient and wanted the patient to be well. But she also wanted to accede to the patient's spoken instruction to not be on a ventilator.

The friend convinced me that the patient had been completely serious about not wanting to be on a ventilator. I struggled with a failure on my part: I had not actually said the words, "You may be on a ventilator after surgery" when I obtained the surgical consent from the patient. I got consent for surgery "and all required post-operative care." Yes, I was in a hurry to explain and get consent because of the patient's waxing and waning consciousness. But to be honest, it never crossed my mind to say, "and you may be on a ventilator."

Ultimately, that evening, after a long and emotional discussion with the friend, and against the will of the hospital administrator, I turned off the ventilator. The patient quickly stopped breathing and died.

There were no consequences. No lawsuit. No reprimand from the administration. Just a terrible feeling that I could have done more. I could have been more thorough in explaining the post-op course when getting the consent.

Would the patient still have signed consent had I mentioned the ventilator? I'll never know. She was in a lot of pain and very frightened. She may have. But she may not have.

Were the ER doctor and nurse admonished? I'll never know that, either.

A Dirty Trick

I was on afternoon rounds with two family practice interns who were both assigned to my surgery service. These young ladies were both very smart and were going to be great family physicians.

Neither of them had any previous military experience and neither was a pilot.

I had been flying the F-16 with my Guard Unit the day before and had pulled a lot of Gs (each G is one force of gravity—on Earth we experience one G). When flying the F-16 we wore G-suits that surrounded our calves, thighs, and abdomens. When we banked or climbed, increasing the G load on our plane and ourselves, the G-suits would automatically inflate to force blood from our lower extremities and abdomen up to our chest and head to help us keep from losing consciousness—the dreaded G-loc (G-induced loss of consciousness).

The G-suits did not cover our chests, buttocks, or upper extremities, and certainly did not cover our necks or heads. Consequently, after flying a high-G flight one would have G-rash everywhere the G-suit did not cover. G-rash was broken capillaries under the skin, which caused red blotches called petechiae. Look at a fighter pilot's neck, back of the scalp, back, and upper extremities and you will see petechiae.

However, petechiae are also a sign of some diseases, such as Rocky Mountain spotted fever, Lyme disease, or leukemias that reduce platelet counts.

Something came over me when one of the interns asked, "Dr. Rizzo, you look tired today. Are you OK?"

I was tired. Flying high-G aircraft is hard work. But instead of telling the interns I had been in the F-16 the day before, I said, "I really am tired. I don't know what's wrong with me. I had a sudden onset of this fatigue yesterday, and now I have this rash."

I pulled up the sleeve of my white coat and showed them the petechiae on my upper extremities.

"Dr. Rizzo, do you have that anywhere else?"

"Yes, I have it on the back of my head, my neck, my back, and my buttocks. And I'm really tired."

By this time, we had walked to my office, where I had planned to have a short sit-down synopsis of the patients and head home.

Instead, the interns, both looking worried, said, "Dr. Rizzo, please wait for us in your office. We'll be right back."

They ran off to the library while I did some paperwork.

After a short while they came back with blood tubes, syringes, a tourniquet, and worried looks on their faces.

"Dr. Rizzo, we want to draw some blood from you. We think you may be very sick, and we want to help you if we can."

They were so sincere, I almost—almost—felt bad for pulling their chains.

I sat them down and explained G-rash to them. I told them I was just kidding them, and they didn't have to worry about me.

They seemed more irritated than relieved. In fact, I suspect they never forgave me.

Sad Truths

After achieving my Air Force retirement goal of living near Walt Disney World and teaching surgery in a civilian residency, why did I quit the residency?

Here's what happened…

Soon after I arrived at the residency, a community surgeon visited me. He told me his surgical group (we'll call them The Big Surgical Practice) had, for several years, been allowing the program's residents to rotate with them. Now that I had been hired by the residency, The Big Surgical Practice was told the residents would no longer rotate with them. He stated the residents slowed down the surgeons and contributed essentially nothing to patient care. But, up to the time of my hiring, The Big Surgical Practice got all the surgical patients from the residency—the drag of having the residents was more than offset by the money earned from the surgical patients.

He then asked, "Have you wondered why it was so easy for you to get this job? Why was Disney and the Celebration project able to arrange for this job without even asking you if you were interested? Why you were hired?"

Good questions.

The answer, he said, was that Medical Center A, one of two competing massive medical center groups (the other we'll call Medical Center B) in the area, had been on a buying spree. It was buying as many practices as it could, of all specialties, to own the medical market in the community and make as much money as possible. Medical Center A had tried, repeatedly, to buy The Big Surgical Practice, but the surgeons were not selling.

"You," he said, "have been hired to force us to sell. Now that all the surgical patients that were being sent to us will go to you, we will lose a significant percentage of our income. You are being used to either drive us out of business or force us to sell our practice to Medical Center A."

I didn't believe him. How could I? I had left my career in the Air Force, which I loved, for what sounded like my retirement dream. How could I believe I was there simply for Medical Center A's political and financial goals? But he was telling the truth. Over the next year-plus, I confirmed that sad truth.

Soon after his visit to my office, two different residents visited me separately. Each told me the same story: I was being badly used because I was *not a member of the religious sect* that owned and administered Medical Center A. Both residents were non-practicing members of the religion. One went so far as to say, "Since you are not a member of their religion, they feel they can do anything they want with you because you are a heathen."

Again, this was so unlike anything I had ever imagined that I didn't believe them. Again, I was wrong.

I was immediately dis-invited from the Celebration hospital planning group when I questioned earmarking several million dollars for a symbol of the religion as part of the construction.

Over the next few months, I learned that I was the only faculty person who was not a member of the religion. I learned that only a few non-members of the religion were accepted to the residency—just sufficient to avoid violating federal anti-discrimination laws.

Not only was I the only non-religion faculty member, I was the only surgeon on the residency faculty. Thus, I was on call every single night for one year, and was called around the clock. I was operating day and night and booking massive billings for the residency.

When I made a point to the residency director about my being on call every night, he promised to hire another surgeon at my one-year anniversary.

I was on a fixed salary and received nothing additional for the surgeries I performed. Over the first year, I discovered my salary was one-fourth that of a family practitioner who only taught in the clinic, did not admit patients, and never was on call. But she was a member of Medical Center A's religion.

I learned I was making one-sixth the salary of the obstetrician/ gynecologists who were members of Medical Center A's religion.

When I discussed with the residency director the financial discrepancies I had discovered, especially given the large amount I was earning for the residency, he was visually upset that I had found out. He actually turned red and stammered. When he recovered his equanimity, he told me I could expect a major raise when my contract was due for renewal at the one-year mark.

He also said everyone in the residency would get a Christmas bonus, and I could expect mine to be significant.

Christmas came. The intern I had rotating on surgery with me was the single worst resident I had ever seen. She was basically ignorant—I had no idea how she got through medical school. But she was a member of the religion. She got a $300 bonus. I got a $6.51 bonus.

I asked the residency director about it. He stated they ran out of money, so my bonus was only $6.51. But I could expect a major raise when he renewed my contract.

At my one year anniversary, the hospital administrator called me into his office to discuss my contract and salary. As soon as the meeting started, he was called out of his office for some reason. On his desk, plainly apparent, were all the contracts for the residency faculty. I took advantage of him being called out to look at some of the contracts. The religion's members were getting massive raises and making many, many times what I was earning.

My contract had no raise.

The administrator returned. Maintaining a straight face, I waited to see what he would say, now knowing what my new contract was to be.

He told me—and this is an exact quote: "Tony, I spoke with God last night. He told me not to give you a raise. He also told me not to hire another surgeon. You will continue to teach surgery by yourself."

I had brought significant surgical case dollars to the residency. Under my instruction, the family practice residents' scores had doubled on the surgery portion of their national in-training exam. The residents had voted me Faculty Member of the Year. But I was the wrong religion, and, most importantly, Medical Center A had been unsuccessful in using me to force The Big Surgical Group to sell to them. Medical Center A had no more use for me.

I left his office, realizing I could no longer work for Medical Center A. I would not continue to teach surgery in this civilian residency.

Now I had to deal with some harsh realities.

There was such animosity between Medical Center A and Medical Center B that I could not be hired by Medical Center B. I know, because I tried.

Joining an established surgical practice meant becoming the junior member of the practice. In surgery, junior practice members are usually given two- or three-year contracts, are not made partners, and have to prove themselves by taking excessive night call while covering weekends and holidays. Usually, at the end of their contracts, the junior members are not offered partnerships. The group usually cuts them loose and finds a new junior member to be their lackey for the next two or three years. Joining an established surgical practice was a no go.

Starting a new solo practice was financially impossible. One has to book, *and collect*, more than twice the cost of the office, staff, and malpractice insurance simply to pay for all of those things plus pay income tax on those earnings. At that time, I would be looking at booking and collecting over a quarter of a million dollars to cover the cost of opening a solo practice—and that didn't include a salary for myself. I would have to find a bank willing to loan me that amount of money, and I did not intend to immerse myself and my family in that level of debt.

I had to face the facts. My surgery days were over.

When I entered the civilian world from Air Force active duty, I was incredibly naïve. Then I lived by, and still live by, the core values of the Air Force: *integrity first, service before self, and excellence in all we do*. I found out the civilian world does not live by those core values.

While teaching surgery at Medical Center A, I had been supervising the residents who were moonlighting on weekends at Walt Disney World's Health Services. I approached Disney, and, fortunately, Disney took me on full time. Which led to my writing *Doctor to the Mouse: Stories from a Walt Disney World Physician*.

Then, 9/11 happened.

That was September 2001. By February 2002, I was back on Air Force active duty, but in Intelligence, not surgery. I stayed on active duty for the next eleven years, until my mandatory Air Force retirement in 2013—yup, I got to be too old to be on active duty.

My kids were adults. My wife and I considered Central Florida our home. We returned there.

Now, I had only memories of surgery.

Afterword

I loved being a surgeon and performing surgery. I loved my time in the Air Force. I loved my time teaching physician assistant students and residents.

But one never really knows what life will bring.

Today, I am retired from surgery and am happily teaching anatomy and physiology at a state college. My students are pre-meds, nurses, physical therapists, occupational therapists, radiographers, and cardiovascular technicians.

In 2015, I received a telephone call from a former patient that prompted this story to be published on the website of my college (used with permission):

25 Years Later, a Phone Call Reunites a Surgeon and a Patient

Posted on Thursday, November 12, 2015 by Polk Newsroom

Two days before Veterans Day, Polk State College Biology Professor Dr. Tony Rizzo's office phone rang.

He was about to head into class. He didn't have much time to spare. But he picked it up anyway.

On the other end of the line was [former patient's name], calling to thank him for saving his life.

"As a surgeon, you never expect to hear from patients again. After this many years, for someone to look me up, I was

humbled and honored that he went to that much trouble," Rizzo said.

In June 1990, [former patient's name], now 72 and living in Las Vegas, was a civilian working for the U.S. Air Force at Lajes Air Force Base in the Azores, a group of islands off the coast of Portugal. On June 8 of that year, [former patient's name] fell gravely ill and required emergency surgery for diverticulitis, a condition that affects the large intestine and causes inflammation, infection and extreme pain.

Rizzo, who came to work at Polk State after retiring as director of the National Center for Medical Intelligence, was stationed at Lajes at the same time, working as the surgeon and chief of hospital services. When [former patient's name] needed surgery, it was Rizzo who came to his aid.

[Former patient's name] explained in an email to News@Polk that Rizzo removed part of his colon and reattached what remained to his small intestine.

"I was full of infection," [former patient's name] wrote.

Rizzo concurred, explaining that [former patient's name] was "full of blood, puss and stool" on the operating table.

"He would have been dead within hours," Rizzo said.

Instead, [former patient's name] went on to make a full recovery. Aside from having surgery to remove a melanoma tumor 10 years ago, he has been healthy ever since.

In the decades that have passed, [former patient's name] has often thought about Rizzo.

"I remember his extreme knowledge of medicine. He was no-nonsense, very serious about his job. He showed great concern for his patients. He was highly respected at Lajes Airfield," [former patient's name] wrote.

Recently, [former patient's name] searched for Rizzo on the Internet. When he came across a 2013 News@Polk article about Rizzo, [former patient's name] was excited to have finally located the man he remembered as "the super surgeon."

"I'm 72 years old and seeing many friends and acquaintances with medical issues. A friend of my daughter's just had a complete hysterectomy, which is probably cancerous. My next-door neighbor and wife are going to the doctor at least once a week. Knock on wood, I am doing OK. I had a flashback to the Azores, on how I almost died 25 years ago. If Dr. Rizzo had not performed this innovative surgery, I would not be writing this. Basically, I just wanted to let him know how grateful I was," [former patient's name] wrote in his email.

When he called Rizzo on Monday, [former patient's name] had a simple aim. He wanted Rizzo to know that he's "breathing and thankful."

For Rizzo's part, while he was happy to hear from [former patient's name], he is quick to eschew any personal attention for having helped him.

"My job was to help people," Rizzo said. "My assignment in the Azores was to be the surgeon and the chief of hospital services. I was literally just doing my job."

Rizzo would go on to reach the rank of Air Force colonel and earn the National Intelligence Distinguished Service Medal, Intelligence Star, and two Defense Superior Service Medals. He retired to Winter Haven in 2013 and currently teaches Human Anatomy and Physiology, Special Topics in Biology, and Basic Principles of Disease at Polk State Winter Haven.

Then, in August of 2021, I received this email from a former patient:

Dr. Rizzo,

I did a search on the web and found where you are. My husband and I wanted to thank you for saving my life at Lajes in 1991. You cleaned up the infection after I had had a hysterectomy. I know that if you had not been the surgeon at Lajes at that time I probably would not have survived. 30 years later and I'm still alive and kicking. Thanks again."

There is no way to express the emotions I felt when those two patients reached out to me.

From time to time someone will ask me if I miss the operating room. I can honestly say that I do not.

I loved Air Force medicine because it was efficient and responsive. If I needed a lab, CT, mammogram, or X-ray I could get it immediately. I didn't have to get approval from an insurance company. My patients always got what they needed.

In the civilian world, medicine is ruled by insurance companies and profit. I simply could not tolerate the kind of restraints that insurance companies place on the civilian doctors I now know and interact with.

I don't envy them at all.

Not to mention, I go home every afternoon, have a three-day weekend every week, get summers off, get a month off around the winter holidays, get spring break and days off for Thanksgiving. Night call is a distant—but unforgotten—memory.

Instead of taking care of one patient at a time I now send 100 or so future doctors, nurses, etc., out into the world every semester. They will take care of legions of patients.

So, I'm content.

About the Author

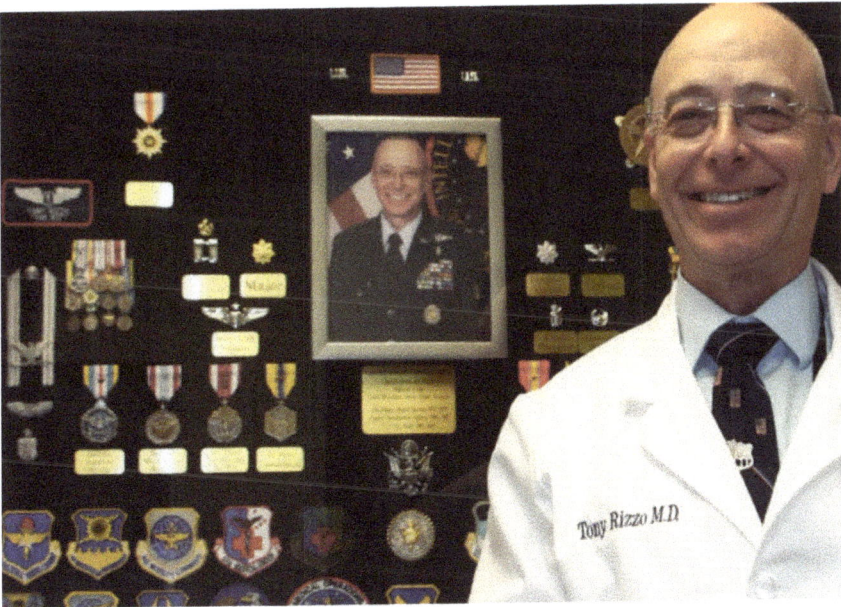

Anthony M. Rizzo, M.D. is dual-trained as a General Surgeon and Aerospace Medicine Physician with thousands of peacetime and wartime surgeries. He retired from the US Air Force after 39 1/2 years of federal service.

CIA Intelligence Officer

Also an Intelligence Officer, he started his career as a CIA officer and ended his career as the Director of the National Center for Medical Intelligence, one of five National Intelligence Centers under the Defense Intelligence Agency. In no particular order, he has either lived or worked in Kinshasa, Zaire (now the Democratic Republic of Congo), Dar es Salaam, Tanzania, every other sub-Saharan African country, Lajes, Azores, Pisa, Italy, Britain, France, Spain, Belgium, the Netherlands, Germany, Switzerland, Greece, Denmark, Iraq, Ukraine, Russia, Romania, Turkey, Sweden, Norway, Finland, Israel, and Egypt.

U.S. Air Force Chief of Surgical Services and Chief of Hospital Services

In the U.S. Air Force Colonel Rizzo was the Chief of Surgical Services and the Chief of Hospital Services at the USAF Hospital, Lajes, Azores. He was a staff surgeon at the USAF Hospital, U.S. Air Force Academy. Colonel Rizzo commanded a 250-bed aeromedical staging squadron (USAF's largest) at Patrick Air Force Base, Florida. After 9/11 he was named the first director of the Surgeon General's Think Thank for Homeland Defense at Brooks City Base, San Antonio, Texas. Colonel Rizzo was the plank-holder (first) Chief of Operations for the Office of the Surgeon General, U.S. Northern Command, Peterson Air Force Base, Colorado Springs, Colorado, as well as for the North American Aerospace Defense Command (NORAD). He then was named the Deputy Command Surgeon for both NORTHCOM and NORAD. He was the Director of the Armed Forces Medical Intelligence Center and converted that organization to the National Center for Medical Intelligence, both under the Defense Intelligence Agency.

Director of National Center for Medical Intelligence

As Director of the National Center for Medical Intelligence Colonel Rizzo oversaw the daily preparation and delivery of intelligence to the President, Vice-President, the Cabinet, the House and Senate, the senior leaders of all military branches including the Joint Chiefs of Staff, and the senior leaders of all the Nation's organizations that receive intelligence. He has testified in closed session before the House Permanent Select Committee on Intelligence. His routine day included visits to the White House, Capitol Hill, and the E-ring (ring for senior leaders) of the Pentagon.

Air Force Flight Surgeon

Col Rizzo is an Air Force Senior Flight Surgeon who was the investigating flight surgeon on two F-16 class-A losses. He has deployed to five armed conflicts. He has logged military flight time in the F-16B, B-1B, KC-135, various C- and KC-130 models, T-37, and the HH-60 helicopter. He was a Space Shuttle Flight Surgeon for seven years.

He is an instrument-rated single-engine land, sea and rotary wing private pilot and has 2,000 hours of civilian pilot-in-command time. He owns and regularly flies a Velocity. His civilian flight time includes over 1200 hours in Velocities, the rest in multiple Cessnas, Pipers, Beechcrafts, Mooneys, the SGS sailplane, and the Ryan PT-22.

Service Medals

Col Rizzo was decorated thirty-seven times; his decorations include the National Intelligence Distinguished Service Medal from the Director of National Intelligence, the Intelligence Star for Valor from the Director of the CIA, two Defense Superior Service Medals and the Defense Meritorious Service Medal from two Secretaries of Defense.

Currently...

Col Rizzo is now a Professor of Anatomy and Physiology at Polk State College in Winter Haven.

An avid woodworker and photographer, his pieces are displayed in museums, galleries, libraries, and cities hall around Central Florida.

He authored *Doctor to the Mouse: Stories from a Walt Disney World Physician*, published by High Tide Publications, Inc. and available on Amazon.com

He is also the author of multiple medical journal articles and textbook chapters.

For more about Col Rizzo's retirement, please see the photographs on the following pages.

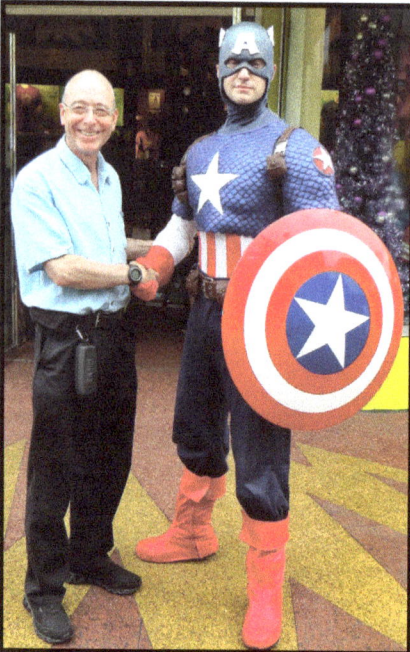

My family took me to meet Captain America at Universal Studios Orlando right after my Air Force retirement.

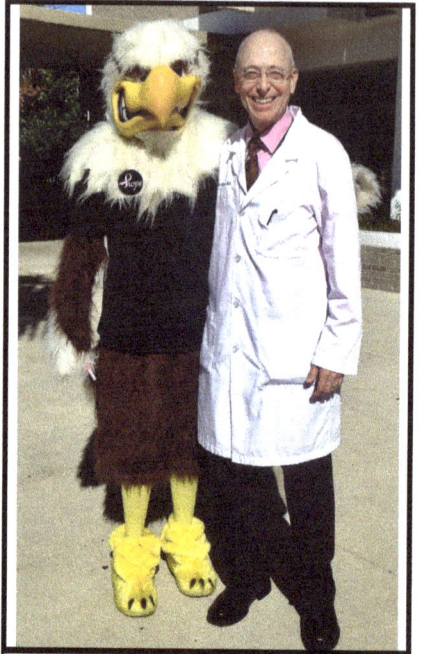

With Charlie, the mascot of the college where I teach Anatomy and Physiology.

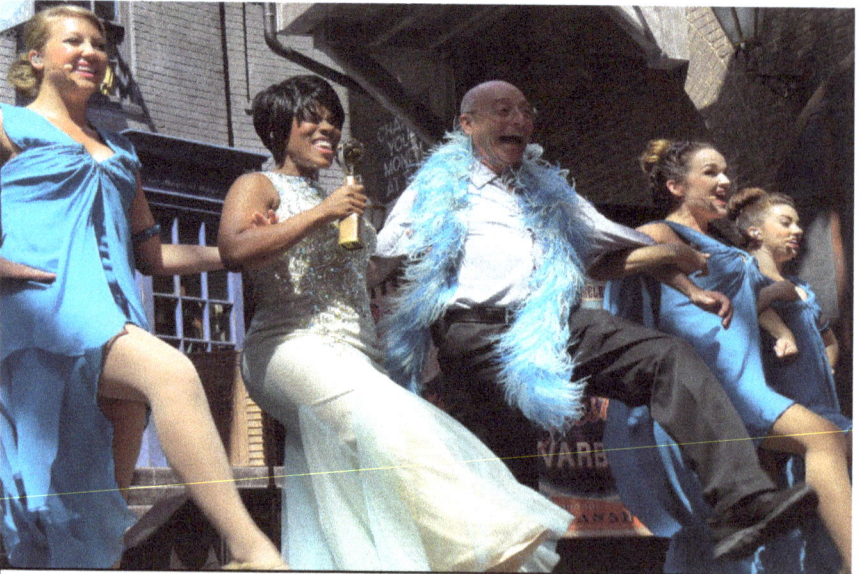

Dancing with Celestina Warbeck and the Banshees in Diagon Alley, Universal Studios Orlando.

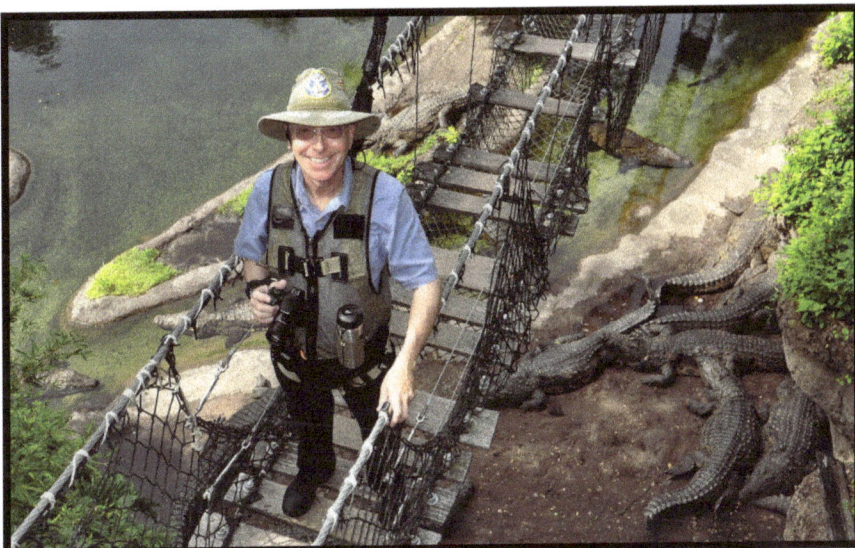

On a backstage tour of Disney's Animal Kingdom, remembering *when you are up to your crack in crocodiles it's difficult to remember that your initial objective was to drain the swamp.*

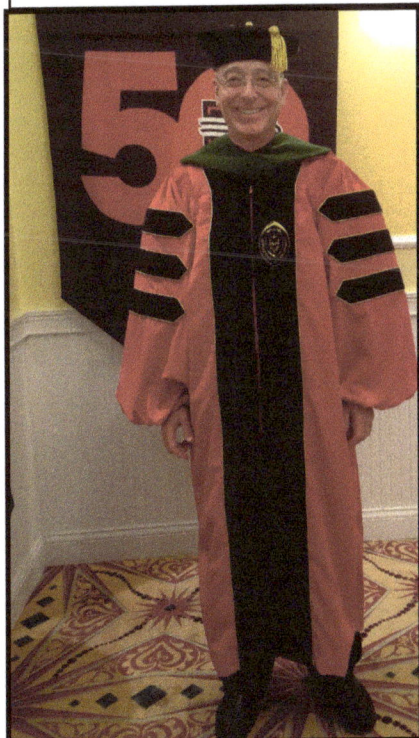

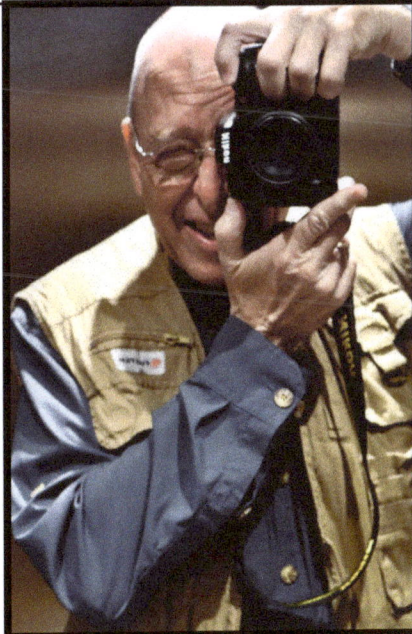

Self-portrait while cruising with my family aboard the *Disney Fantasy.*

In academic regalia at a graduation ceremony at Polk State College in Winter Haven.

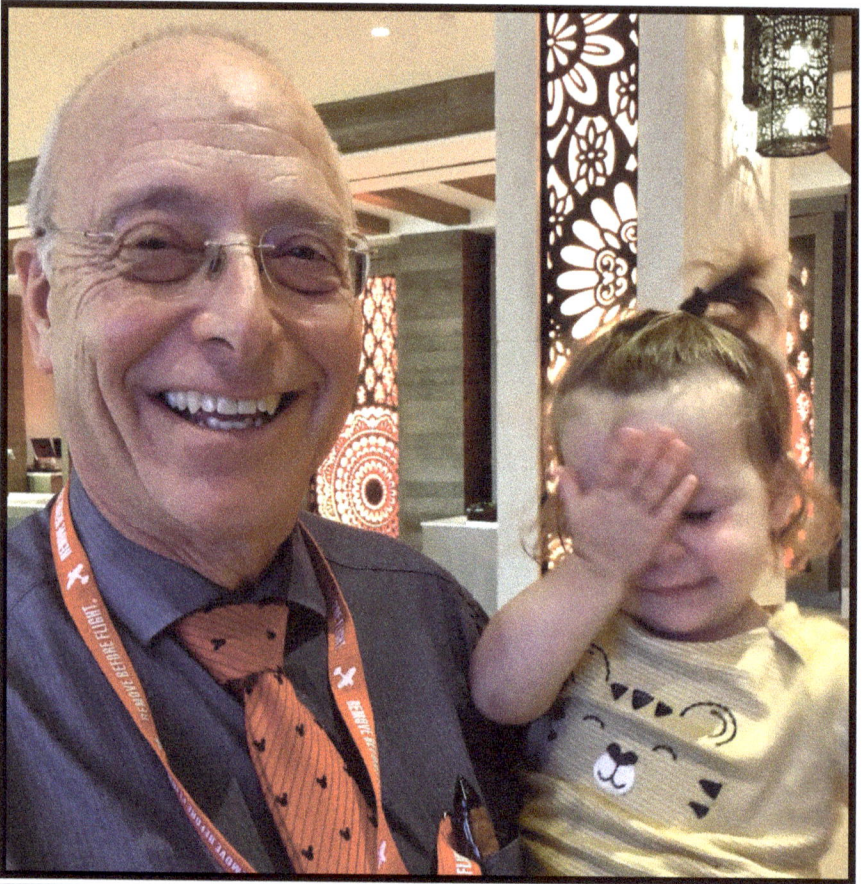

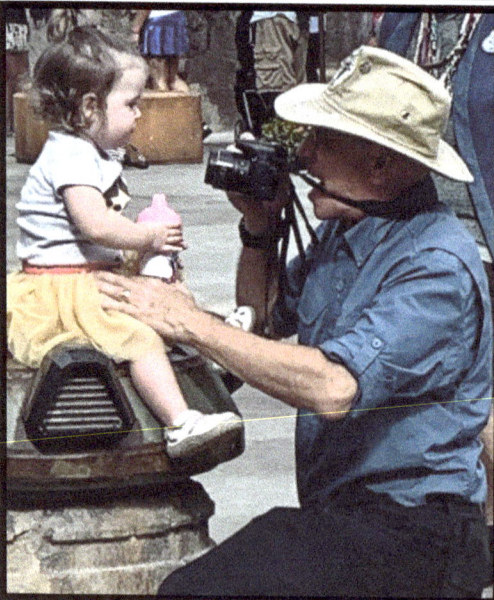

Above:

My granddaughter's dad joke response.

Left:

With my granddaughter on the planet Batuu at the opening of *Star Wars: Galaxy's Edge* in Disney's Hollywood Studios.

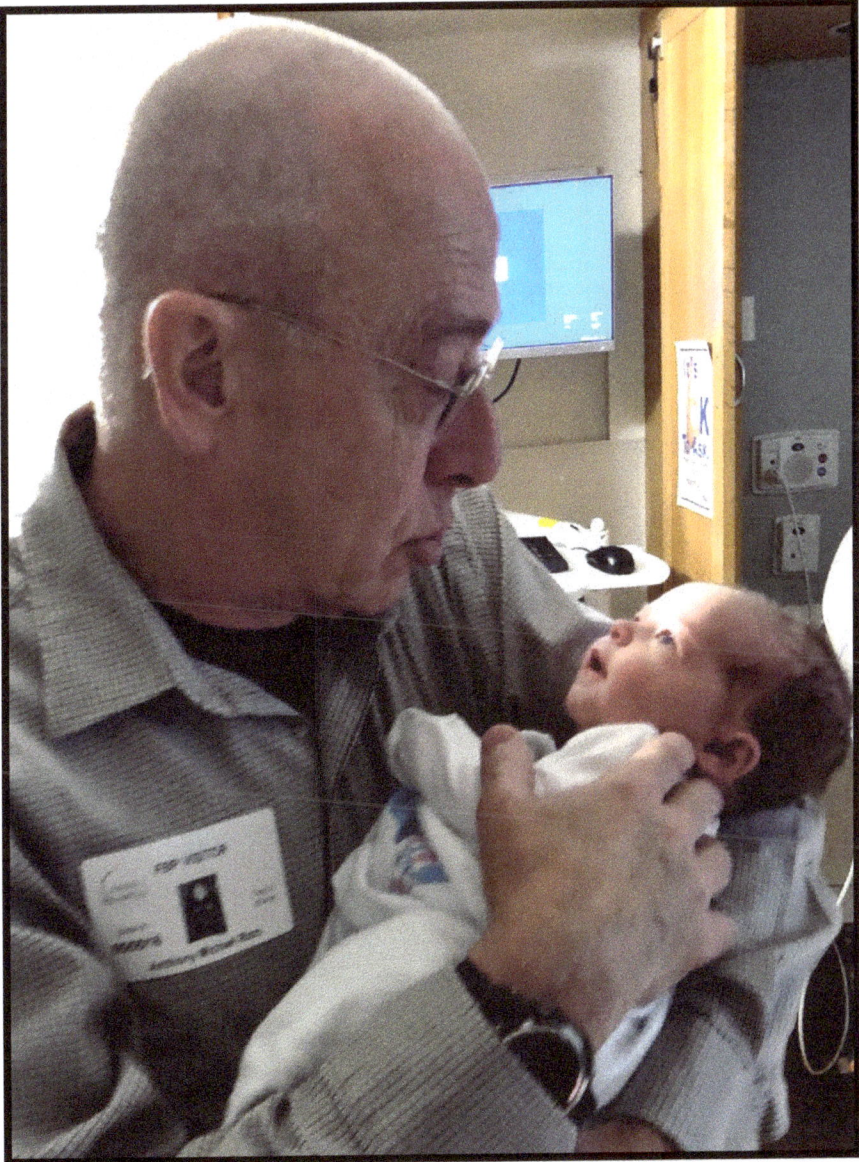

Meeting my first grandchild

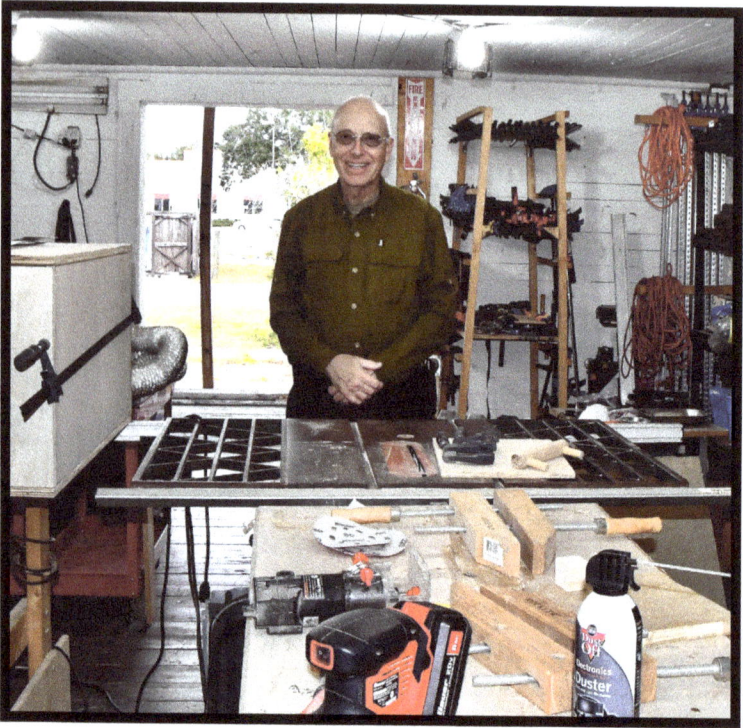

In my woodworking shop.

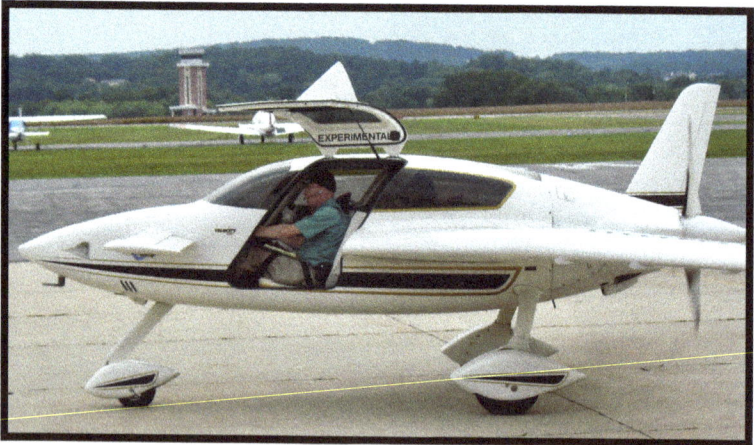

Preparing for take-off in my Velocity airplane.

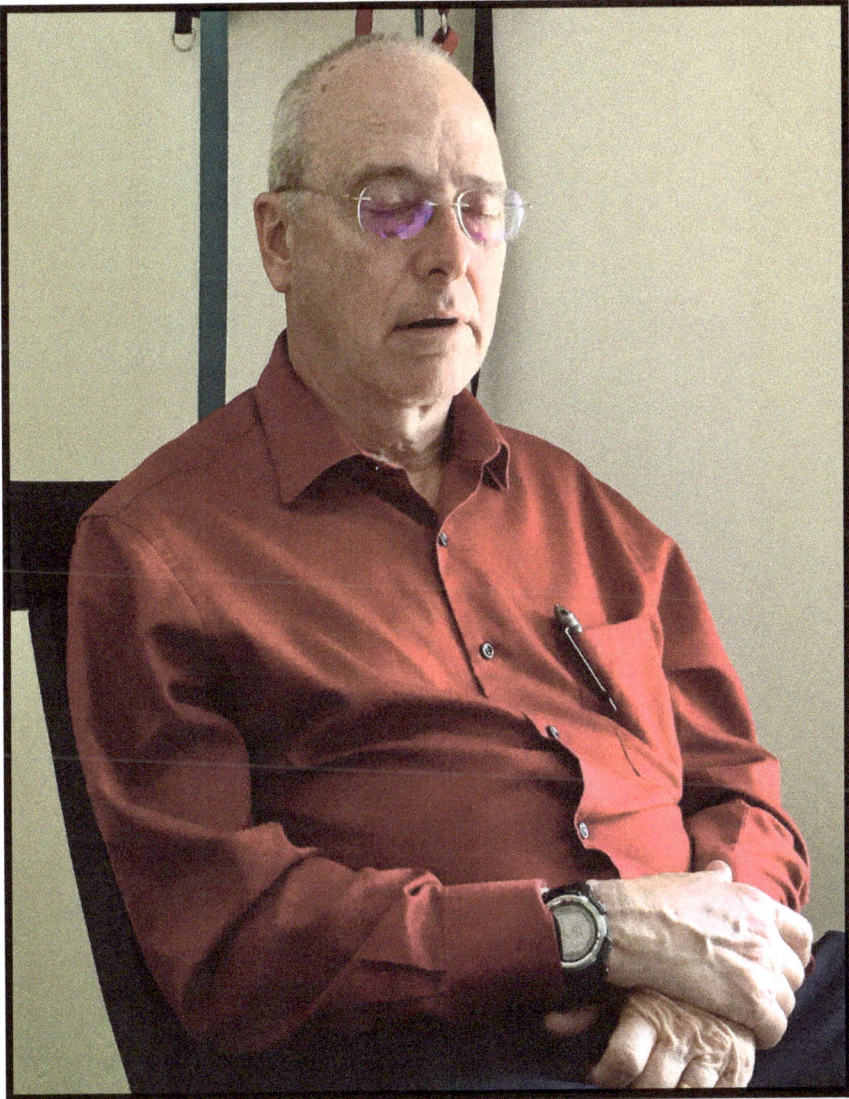

Semper vigilate! Ever alert! The Intelligence Officer's hallmark...

Acknowledgments

To every patient who trusted me with their health and life over my training and practice years: there are no words sufficient to thank you

To every nurse who took care of my patients over the years: you are the true heroes of medicine

To my students: you are the future of medicine. As they said in my surgery training, there are two grades when taking care of patients—'A' and 'F'. 'A' is 100%. 'F' is 99% and below. You are human, but strive for an A

To Jeanne Johansen and Cindy Freeman at High Tide Publications: I thought I wrote an "OK" book. You made it much, much better

Finally, and most importantly, to my wife, children, children-in-law, and grandchildren: It's cliché but true—without you I am nothing

A Note From the Publisher

The world of medicine has changed drastically since the days Tony Rizzo attended medical school in the 1970s and 1980s. We hope, if you are reading this book, and thinking about joining the medical profession, please know the world needs you. The fight to save lives remains the same.

If this glimpse into Dr. Rizzo's experiences school resonated with you, we would would be grateful for your review.

Sharing your thoughts helps keep these stories alive and ensures the history of how surgeons were forged is not forgotten.

Thank you from all of us at High Tide Publications, Inc.

www.ingramcontent.com/pod-product-compliance
Lightning Source LLC
Chambersburg PA
CBHW041930090426
42744CB00017B/2000